To Ralph—

A great dentist and contemporary — with whom it is a pleasure to share our profession!

Buddy Frumm

OCCLUSAL TREATMENT

OCCLUSAL TREATMENT

Preventive and Corrective Occlusal Adjustment

NORMAN R. ARNOLD, D.D.S., M.Sc.

SANFORD C. FRUMKER, D.D.S.

School of Dentistry
Case Western Reserve University
Cleveland, Ohio

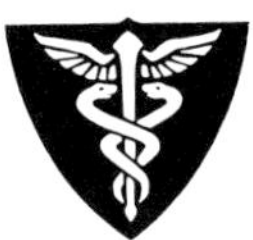

LEA & FEBIGER · 1976 · PHILADELPHIA

Library of Congress Cataloging in Publication Data

Arnold, Norman R
  Occlusal treatment.

  Bibliography: p.
1. Occlusion (Dentistry)   I. Frumker, Sanford C.,
joint author.   II. Title.   [DNLM: 1. Dental
occlusion.   2. Malocclusion—Therapy.   3. Orthodontics.
WU440 A757o]
RK523.A76   1975   617.6′43   75-1306
ISBN 0-8121-0526-5

Published in Great Britain by Henry Kimpton Publishers, London
Printed in the United States of America

Dedicated to

The memory of my father, Carl C. Arnold...(nra) Dick Lurie and Manuel Lopez Ramos, two of the finest teachers and greatest human beings I have ever known . . . . (scf)

PREFACE

This book was written because we believe much needs to be said about occlusion. In harking back to early dentistry and to our own educational experience, we note that the major battles in the area of occlusion were waged on the wrong front: the disaster front. Every occlusal disaster must have had a beginning, and occlusal treatment at the beginning probably would have prevented the disaster.

Discussions of techniques for handling occlusal disaster or fullmouth bridgework or full dentures do not appear in this work. The subject is how to place restorations that build a resistant occlusion, and how to grind or adjust teeth for occlusal health. Of course, the occlusal disaster is considered here, but most of the text applies to occlusal treatment of the average dental patient. The procedures described can be performed by every dentist, and at a fee the patient can accept. Furthermore, the treatment is preventive.

Our discussion is limited to the everyday, clinical practice problems of occlusal treatment. No attempt is made to teach anatomy, physiology, or other basic sciences.

It is our intent to provide the reader with an in-depth feeling for, and understanding of, the principles of occlusion, and to help provide him with the abilities:

(1) to apply the principles to routine restorative dentistry;
(2) to examine for and detect occlusal disease or traumatism and to prevent it;
(3) to perform a complete occlusal adjustment by selective grinding;
(4) to recognize the completeness and correctness of such an adjustment,

and then, when he has had experience and success in tightening loose teeth, stopping habitual bruxing, and effecting lasting healthy occlusions—he will more confidently do occlusal treatment, and become more aware of the important role occlusion plays in periodontal health.

The principles of occlusion are fundamental, but we expect the practitioner to find more and better ways to apply them.

NORMAN R. ARNOLD

SANFORD C. FRUMKER

Cleveland, Ohio

OUR THANKS TO:

The great group of people with whom we had contact during our formative years, and who gave us so much: John R. Wilson, our great teacher at Ohio State Dental College; and Steven W. Brown.

All our students at Case Western Reserve University Dental School—both undergraduate and postgraduate—from whom *we* have learned so much.

Our fellow faculty members at Case Western Reserve University Dental School.

A very special thanks to Dr. Charlie Sellnau, our close friend, who spent hours reviewing our manuscript and making suggestions.

The many meetings and discussions with our 15 fellow members of the Cleveland Academy for Preventive Dentistry.

All the past and present greats in occlusion with whom we have had no personal communication, but whose writings and ideas contributed so much to ours. To even begin to list them all is impossible.

The Department of Research in Medical Education (DORIME) of Case Western Reserve University who pre-published and tested this book.

Marv Lockman, our artist.

Our secretary, receptionist, typist, book-keeper, confidant, and protector, Miss Gloria Perlberg.

Lea and Febiger, and especially Mary Mansor, for their help and cooperation.

CONTENTS

1

Occlusal Treatment Is Unavoidable

The term *occlusion* refers to the way that teeth touch each other. Faulty occlusion results in disease, which can be prevented or eliminated only by dental treatment.

Occlusal change, or alteration in the occluding surfaces of opposing teeth, is a never-ending process. It begins when the teeth touch each other during the eruption process and is carried on, by the patient and by the dentist, continuously throughout life. Either optimal or damaging force is applied to the teeth by the contacts they make, and occlusal health or occlusal disease results from these contacts.

In the broadest sense, contacts on teeth include occlusal contact (between opposing teeth), proximal contact (between adjacent teeth), and contact with the tongue, lips, cheeks, foods, prosthetic appliances, and foreign objects. These contacts in themselves are further modified by the habits and environment of the individual patient. Although all the contacts mentioned produce force that can affect health, the most significant contact is that between opposing teeth—occlusal contact.

Facets—shiny flat wear areas—are evidence of occlusal adjustment made by the patient, as are mobility and fremitus. *Fremitus* is the vibration or slight movement of an upper tooth that occurs when the patient taps or rubs his teeth together. It can be felt by the examiner if he places his fingertip on both the gingiva and the facial surface of the upper tooth simultaneously (see Fig. 59). A facet opposite a supporting cusp is usually an interference, and the patient, in an effort to eliminate the interference, wears away his supporting cusps. It is an undesirable technique and a waste of tooth structure. Only a dentist can remove the interferences and at the same time preserve the patient's supporting cusps.

MOST DENTISTRY IS OCCLUSAL TREATMENT

We are especially interested in the role of the dentist in occlusal adjustment. Despite the importance attached to occlusion by their instructors, most dental students are unsure, even at graduation, about doing occlusal treatment. They have been told *not* to adjust occlusions preventively, an inconsistent philosophy, since nearly everything they do is essentially occlusal treatment, for better or worse. In other words, the dentist provides occlusal treatment every time he alters the occlusal surface of a tooth, and such routine restorations comprise a major part of his practice. It behooves him, then, consciously to ensure good results by establishing a definite objective for specific occlusal contacts.

OCCLUSAL ADJUSTMENT

Occlusal adjustment is either constructive (preventive) or destructive. It is effected by restorations, selective grinding, orthodontics, or bruxism. There cannot be any question about the need for preventive occlusal treatment since the alternative to it is destructive occlusal treatment.

Let us consider the two aspects of treatment: (1) elimination of occlusal interferences by selective grinding and (2) restoration or, better, the creation of tooth structure with prosthetic materials.

Occlusal interferences can be defined as tooth contacts that interfere with the way a person wants to move or close his jaw. They restrain the patient. Occlusal restraints prevent the mandible from following normal paths of movement or closure and

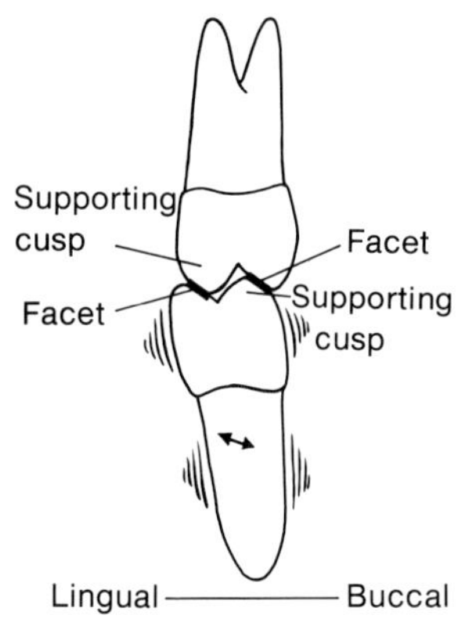

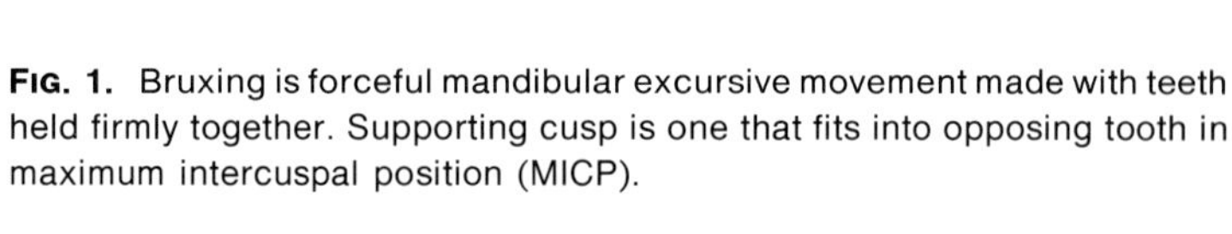
FIG. 1. Bruxing is forceful mandibular excursive movement made with teeth held firmly together. Supporting cusp is one that fits into opposing tooth in maximum intercuspal position (MICP).

cause occlusal traumatism by inducing bruxing (Fig. 1). During bruxing the cuspal inclines strike and deflect or push the teeth sideward, causing occlusal traumatism. Sometimes it takes years to "knock the tooth out of the way." Sometimes only part of the tooth is worn out of the way, and a facet results.

INTERFERENCES → RESTRAINT → OCCLUSAL TRAUMATISM

Occlusal traumatism is another term for occlusal disease. A serious dental problem, it causes the destruction of the periodontium and, ultimately, the loss of teeth. Occlusal traumatism can be detected clinically. Its cause is force—too much, in the wrong direction (horizontally), and for too long a time. In other words, the force on the teeth either "knocks them in" (resulting in occlusal health) or "knocks them out" (resulting in occlusal traumatism) (Fig. 2).

Occlusal treatment often is discussed in terms of orthodontics, full mouth reconstruction, or occlusal adjustment by selective grinding. In reality, however, occlusion is treated every time a routine restoration involves the occlusal surface of a tooth.

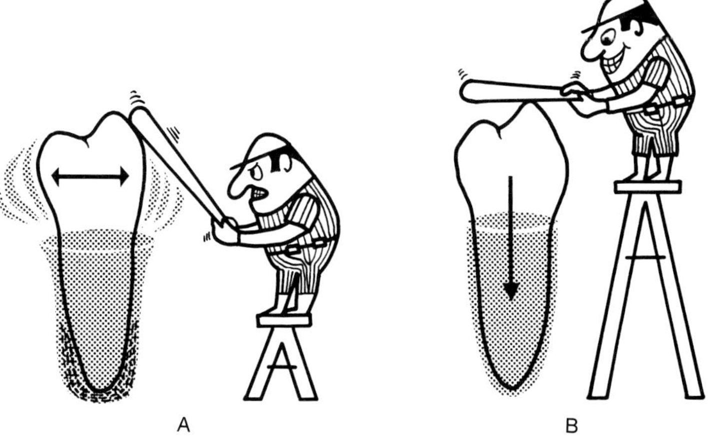

FIG. 2. *A,* Occlusal traumatism (horizontal force). *B,* Occlusal health (axial force).

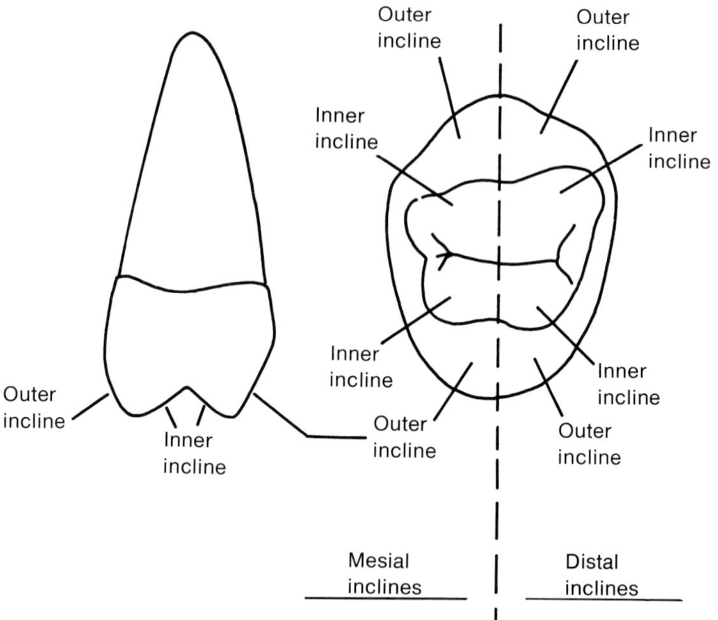

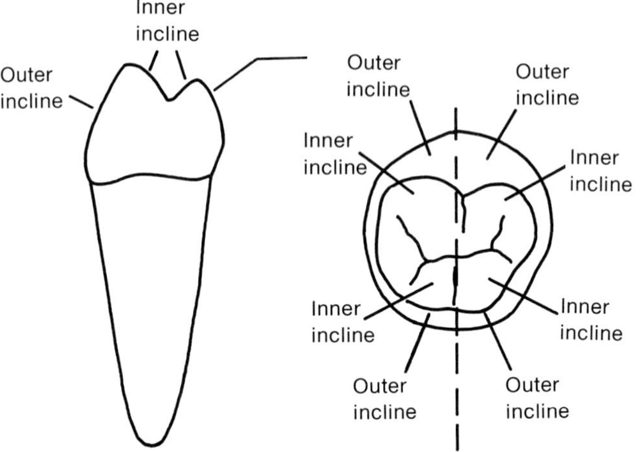

FIG. 3. Each cusp has an inner and outer incline in relation to its tip. Inner incline extends from cusp tip to central groove. Outer incline extends from cusp tip to outer surface of tooth. Cusp tips further divide inner and outer inclines into mesial and distal inclines.

EVERY RESTORATION IS A CREATION FOR THE INDIVIDUAL PATIENT

In any occlusal relationship, how should the restoration contact the opposing tooth? If articulating ribbon is placed between the teeth and the patient is asked to close or rub his teeth together, exactly what kind of markings should be expected? All too frequently, examination reveals markings that defy explanation.

To achieve occlusal contacts that effect a healthy occlusion, the dentist must be guided by specific occlusal contact objectives. Occlusal contacts should result in:

1. *Axial forces* on the teeth

2. *Mandibular stability* (a stable condition in which the muscles can fit the mandible so that it will not slip in relation to the infrahyoid and associated musculature)

3. *Freedom* of the mandible to move to and from the occlusal contacts without interference from cuspal inclines

The achievement of these objectives is the subject of this book. (The names of the cuspal inclines that are used to describe the occlusal surfaces of the teeth are given in Figure 3.)

2

Posterior Tooth Contact: The Cusp Seat

A simple, practical concept in restorative and operative dentistry whose application will result in axial forces, mandibular stability, and freedom is that of the *cusp seat*, the therapeutic replacement of the fossa and marginal-ridge areas of the teeth. The cusp seat consists of three easily formed parts:

1. Pinpoint contact

2. Holding boundary, or reference area

3. Freedom areas

PINPOINT CONTACT

The pinpoint contact is a minute area on the cusp seat at which an opposing cusp tip touches the cusp seat. The pinpoint contact *stops* and *stabilizes* the mandible, providing for efficient functioning of the musculature associated with the mandible. At the same time, it results in *axial forces on the teeth*, thereby promoting occlusal health.

Naturally, for axial loading the long axes of opposing teeth should be nearly in line with or parallel to each other, permitting both teeth to receive axial force on occlusal contact (Fig. 4A). Practically speaking, the long axes between opposing teeth cannot be perfectly in line with each other; but the more nearly in line they are the better. Otherwise, occlusal contacts result in nonaxial force (Fig. 4B) and may require orthodontic treatment.

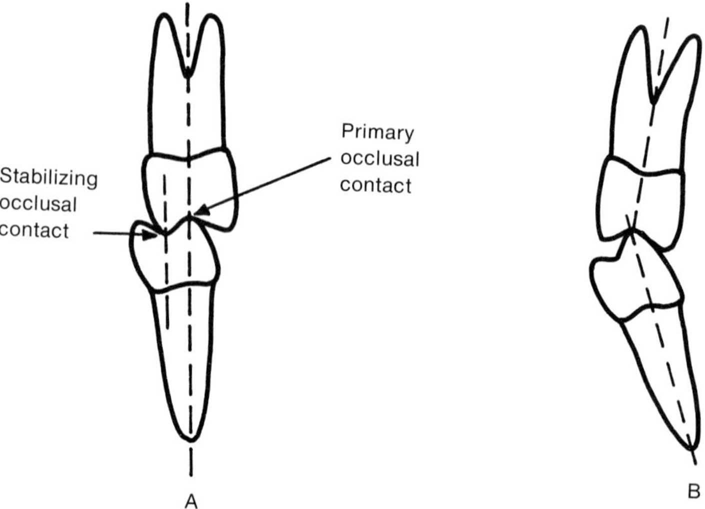

FIG. 4. *A,* Axes are parallel. *B,* Axes are nonparallel.

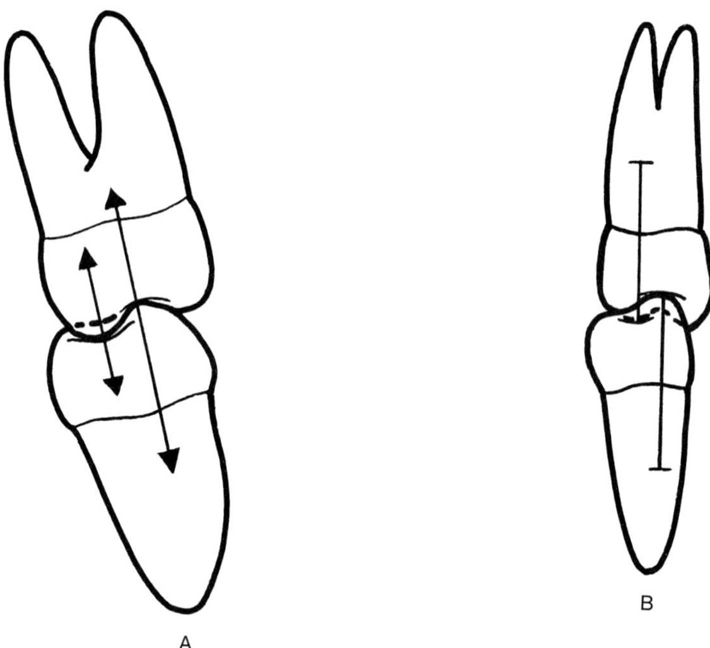

FIG. 5. *A,* Primary and stabilizing occlusal contacts. Primary occlusal contact is between lower buccal cusp and upper fossa. Stabilizing contact is between upper lingual cusp and lower fossa. *B,* Pinpoint occlusal contact.

The main pinpoint occlusal contacts are the primary contact and the stabilizing contact. The *primary contact*, between the lower buccal cusp tip and the opposing upper fossa or marginal-ridge area, is the best for axial loading. The line of force from this contact better approximates the center of the alveoli, or bony housing of the teeth. The *stabilizing occlusal contact*, between the upper lingual cusp tip and lower fossa or marginal-ridge area, joins the primary occlusal contact to stabilize the teeth and prevent tipping (Fig. 5).

The objective is to establish only primary and stabilizing contacts on the teeth. *A fundamental principle of occlusal health is that contact between cuspal inclines should be avoided.* The proximal contacts can also aid in stabilizing the teeth (Fig. 21).

HOLDING BOUNDARY

The holding boundary, or reference area or position, is a slight occlusal rise in the contour of a cusp seat. It is continuous with the pinpoint contact in an upper and lower cusp seat.

The holding boundary prevents the mandible from slipping forward off the pinpoint contact and ensures the stability of the mandible in centric occlusion (Fig. 6A). It also programs the neuromuscular system so that the individual can repeatedly stabilize the mandible with the same cusp tip–cusp seat contacts.

The holding boundary serves as a reference for the neuromuscular system much the same as a door molding can serve as a reference for finding a light switch in a dark room. Every jaw closes to a reference position, which is its most stable position. It is the position that the casts "fit" in when they are handheld.

The casts can be handheld in this maximum intercuspal position without slipping, and, in fact, are held in this position when a wax bite is not available. If the hand muscles find the maximum intercuspal position (MICP) stable, then so do the muscles associated with the jaws. However, if the teeth are not axially loaded in this position, occlusal disease can develop.

The use of cusp seats in restorations insures a reference position that axially loads the teeth.

Holding boundaries (also referred to as centric stops when they occur in centric relation) are sometimes lost on posterior

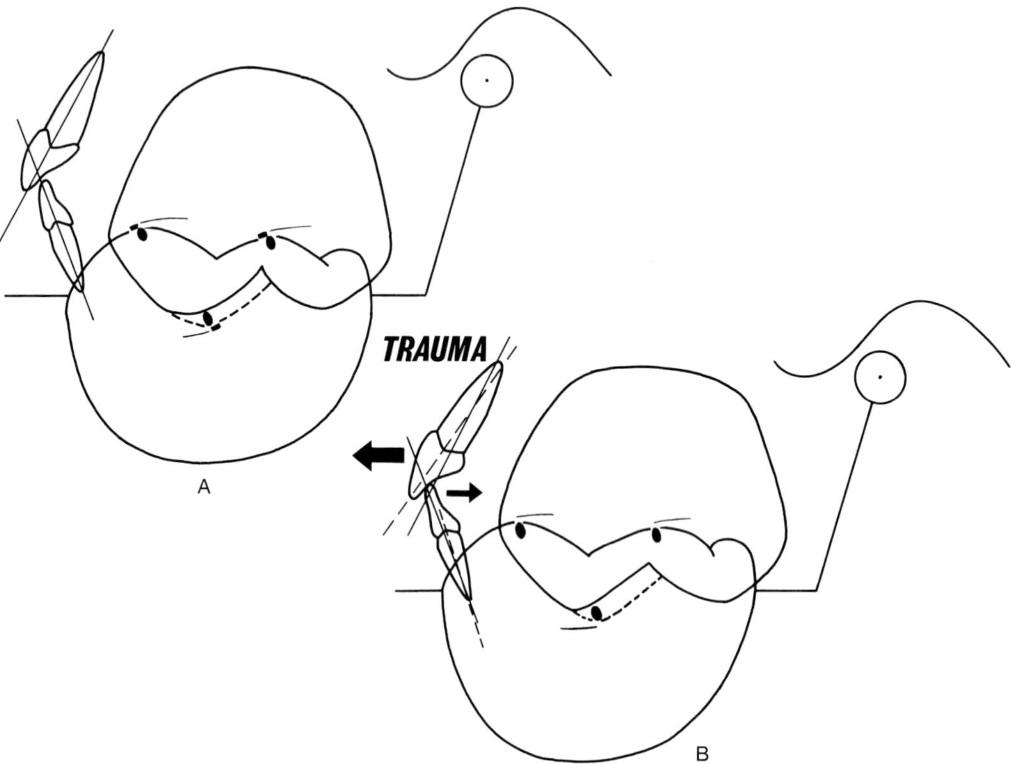

A

B

FIG. 6. **A,** Holding boundary is shown as heavy black line. It is mesial to contact points (*black dots*) on upper tooth and distal to contact point on lower tooth. Mandible is stabilized so that it will not slide forward. **B,** Holding boundary is missing. There is no heavy black line mesial to contact points on upper tooth. Mandible is not stabilized and slides forward, causing restraint of posterior teeth and traumatogenic occlusal contacts on anterior teeth.

teeth, in which case the patient stops and stabilizes his mandible in a more anterior position. This may cause the lower anterior teeth to strike the lingual surfaces of the upper anterior teeth so hard that the upper anterior teeth become flared labially. The patient is then forced to use the anterior teeth as holding boundaries, and the result is occlusal traumatism to the anterior teeth (Fig. 6B).

FREEDOM AREA

The freedom area is the flattened area around the remainder of the pinpoint cusp-seat contact. It provides a multidirectional approach and escape route for an opposing cusp tip. In other words, the freedom area does not interfere with the opposing cusp tip as it moves in and out of the cusp seat (Fig. 7). It extends for one or two millimeters around the pinpoint contact, but it does not extend into the holding boundary.

The mandible is stabilized in the maximal intercuspal position (MICP) when the teeth are occluded. More often than not, the MICP is slightly anterior to centric relation (CR). A freedom area distal to the pinpoint contact in an upper cusp seat affords the patient the option of closing in CR while maintaining axial forces on the teeth. In other words, the teeth can be closed in a more distal relationship (CR) without interference from inclines (Fig. 8).

In a lower cusp seat, the freedom area is mesial to the pinpoint contact, allowing for a more distal positioning of the mandible in centric relation (Fig. 9).

Lack of freedom, referred to as restraint, causes tension in the patient; and to release this tension the patient bruxes. As long as the tension or restraint remains, the patient continues to brux. The bruxing is usually done during sleep, and most people who brux do not know they do it. Bruxing produces very damaging horizontal forces that cause occlusal traumatism.

When the patient bruxes, he uses his supporting cusps to wear away the restraining inclines. Unfortunately, the supporting cusps are worn away faster than the restraining inclines are. In addition, the patient loses mandibular stability in the retruded position as his supporting cusps are worn away.

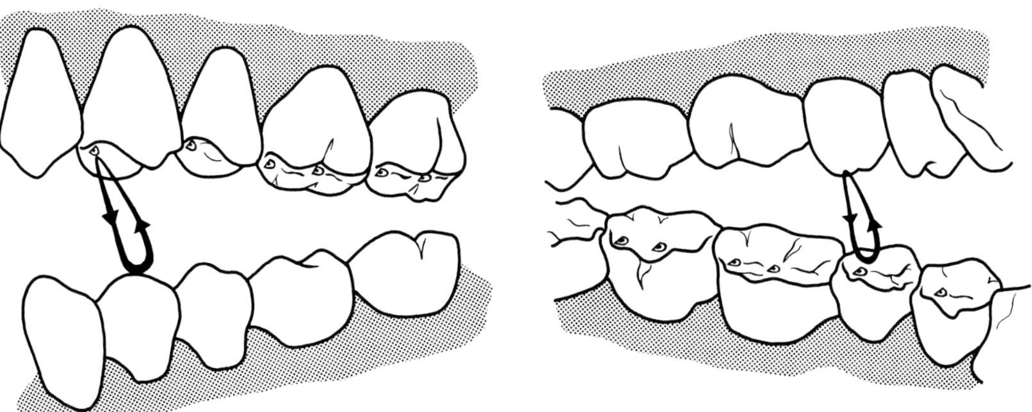

FIG. 7. Cusp seat provides freedom for cusps to move to and from opposing teeth without interferences from cuspal inclines.

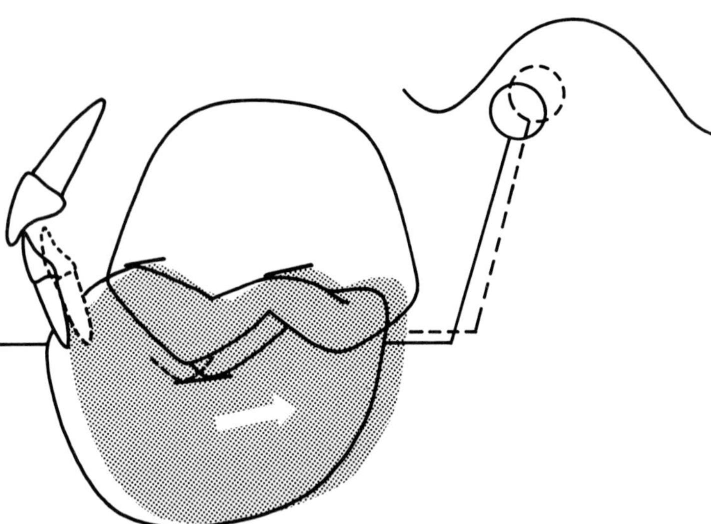

Fig. 8. When maximum intercuspal position (MICP) is anterior to centric relation (CR), freedom area distal to contact point in upper cusp seat and mesial to contact point in lower cusp seat allows patient to close more distally and into centric relation. Without this freedom, move to CR would be blocked by interfering inclines. Solid line shows MICP. Dotted line shows CR position with no interferences because of freedom in cusp seats.

The only way the patient can eliminate occlusal restraint is with an abrasive diet. But modern man does not have an abrasive diet, and therefore it is up to the dentist to treat the problem. This section shows how to place a single restoration so that it will axially load a tooth, contribute to mandibular stability, and not cause restraint. Although treatment and adjustment of the entire occlusion is the subject of this book, here, we will concentrate on the single restoration. Once axial loading, freedom, and stability on a single restoration are achieved, applying it to the entire occlusion will logically follow.

APPLYING THE CUSP-SEAT CONCEPT

There are five types of occlusal contact relationships that the dentist must restore: (1) cusp-to-fossa, (2) cusp-to-marginal-ridge, (3) cusp-to-incline, (4) cusp-to-cusp, and (5) crossbite (Figs. 10, 11).

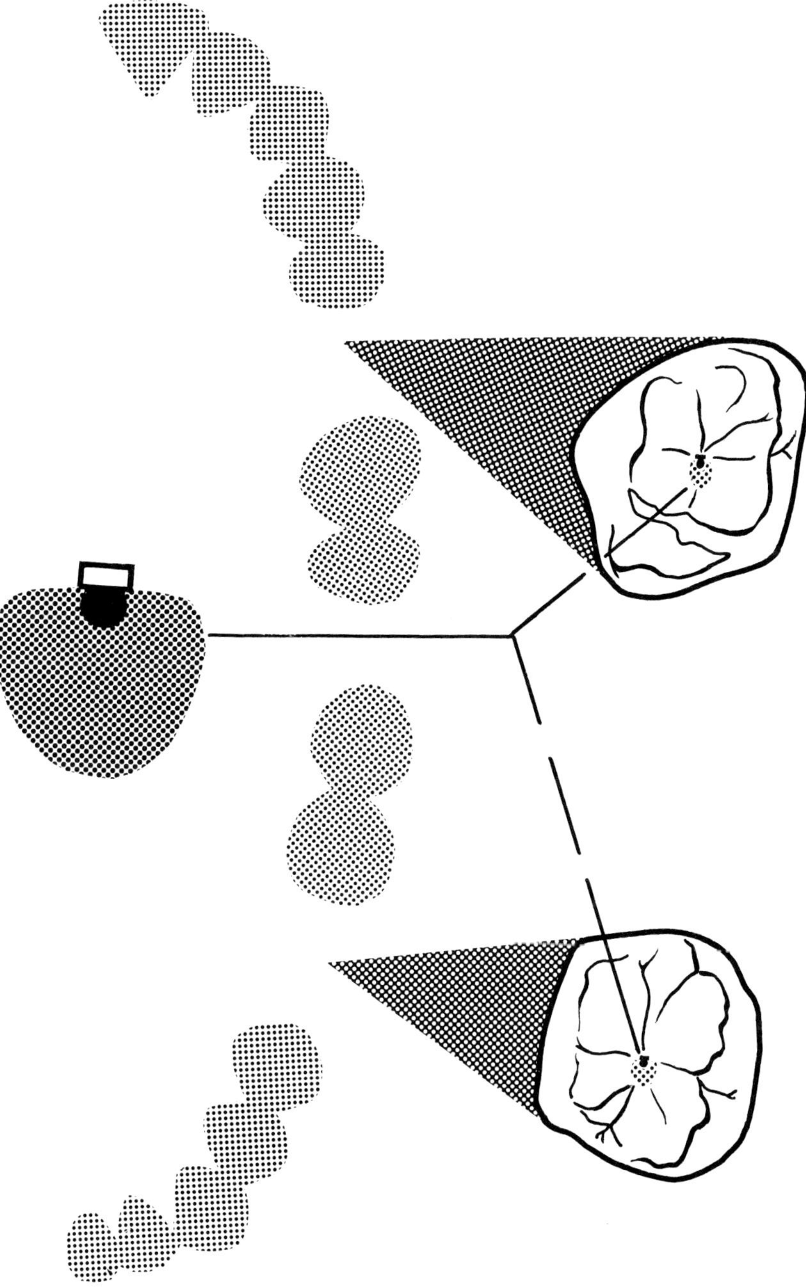

FIG. 9. Black dot represents pinpoint contact dot of cusp seat. Rectangle is holding boundary. Note that in upper molar, holding boundary is mesial to contact dot and in lower molar, distal to contact dot. Dotted area around contact dot represents freedom area. Cusp seat is shown in two first molars to indicate its comparative size.

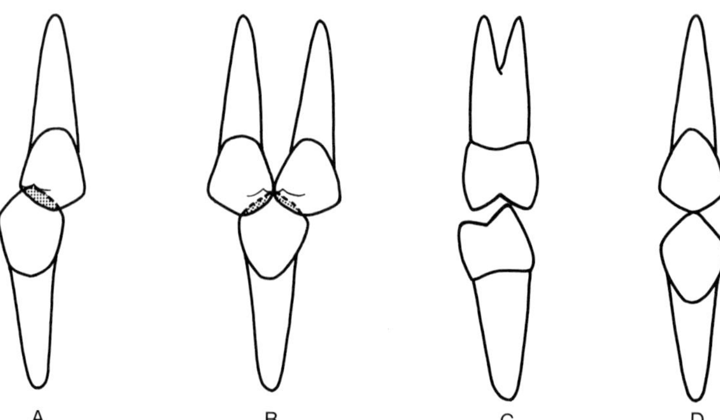

FIG. 10. Types of occlusal contact relationships. *A,* Cusp-to-fossa. *B,* Cusp-to-marginal ridge (embrasure). *C,* Cusp-to-incline. *D,* Cusp-to-cusp.

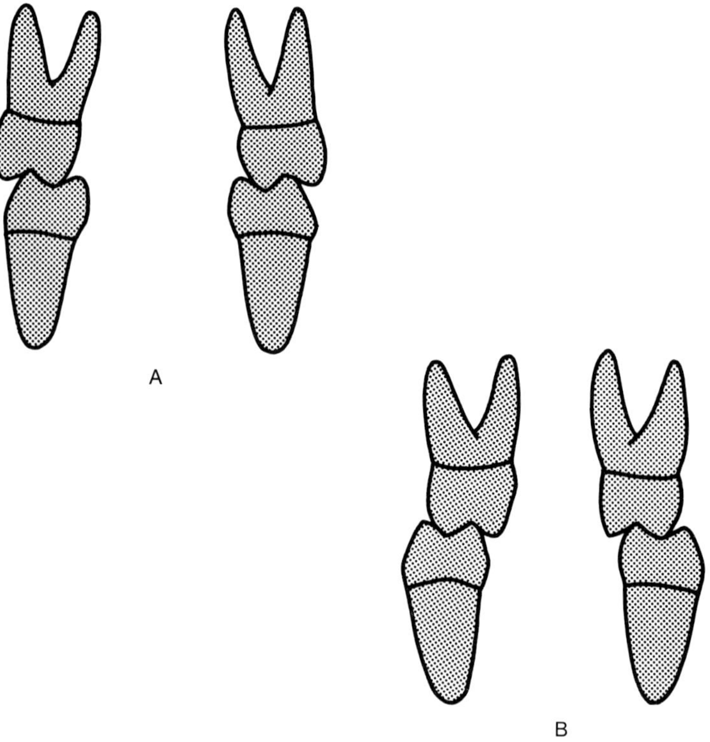

FIG. 11. *A,* Normal occlusal relationships. *B,* Crossbite relationship.

Cusp-To-Fossa Relationship

A cusp-to-fossa relationship exists when a cusp tip is opposite to and within the area of a fossa while the teeth are in occlusion. To restore this relationship, the fossa is therapeutically replaced with a cusp seat. To carve the original fossa anatomy into a restoration, one would have to balance the opposing cusp tip on three or four inclines of the fossa simultaneously. This is impractical if not impossible. The cusp seat, on the other hand, requires only one pinpoint contact, a practical and more easily accomplished goal (Fig. 12C).

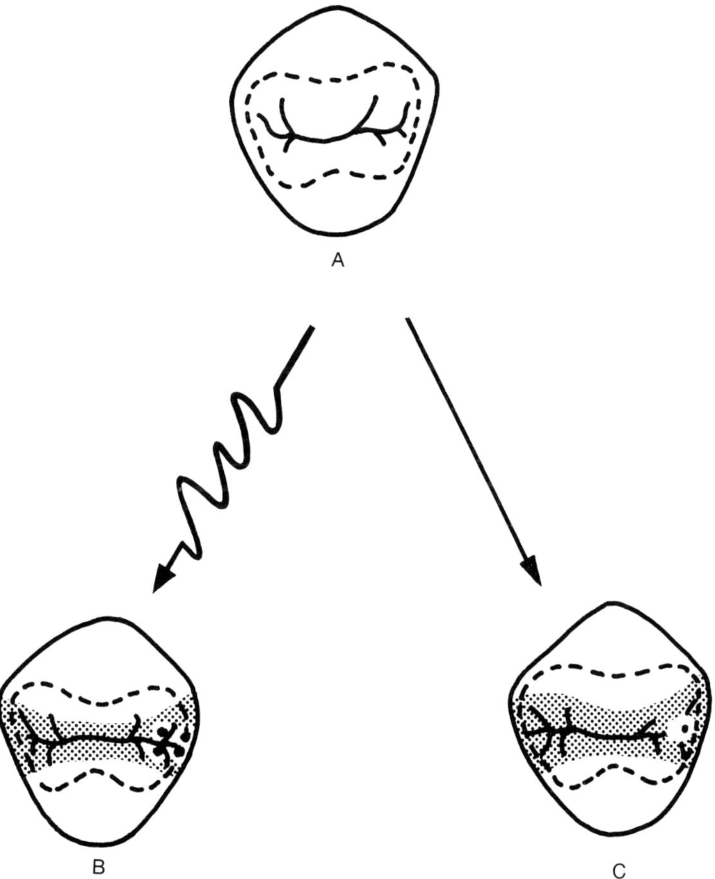

FIG. 12. *A,* Carious tooth. *B,* The hard way, balancing three or four contact points on inclines of fossa. These contacts are shown as four dots around the pit in the fossa. *C,* The practical way, replacing fossa with cusp seat, where there is only one pinpoint contact.

EXAMINATION. Occlusal relationships can be determined from study models, by looking directly into the mouth or by having the patient bite into wax or tap the teeth together on articulating ribbon. The occlusion is examined to determine the location of the opposing cusp tip in relation to the fossa that must be restored. Is it opposite the fossa? Is it between marginal ridges? Is it opposite a cuspal incline? Or is the relationship cusp-to-cusp or crossbite? (See Figs. 10, 11)

For the sake of the immediate discussion, let us suppose that we are dealing with a cusp-to-fossa relationship, the ideal relationship. Whether or not the fossa to be restored has undergone previous restoration is not significant.

TECHNIQUE FOR PLACING CUSP SEAT
(CUSP-TO-FOSSA RELATIONSHIP)

I. Mark the Teeth

Have the patient tap the teeth together on articulating ribbon in the MICP. When using articulating ribbon, be sure the teeth and ribbon are *absolutely dry*. Control excessive salivation (p. 114). While holding the ribbon between the teeth, tell the patient to "chop, chop." This helps him to tap his teeth together rather than chew on the ribbon. You can demonstrate what you want the patient to do by tapping your own teeth together. The object is to have the patient tap his teeth together in the MICP (Fig. 13A).

II. Adjust the Occlusion

Grind away any marks on *cuspal inclines* around the fossa (or fossae) to be restored. Grind away any marks on cuspal inclines on the opposing cusp only if it is severly worn. Do not grind or polish the very tip of the opposing cusp that is opposite the fossa. By the very tip of a cusp, is meant approximately the one millimeter surrounding the peak of the cusp (Fig. 13B).

III. Check the Occlusal Adjustment

Check the occlusal adjustment by repeating Step I. If any marks appear on inclines, they should be polished away as in Step II. When the occlusal adjustment is completed, there will be one of two possible results. One possibility is that the fossa to be restored and the opposing cusp tip contact each other in the MICP so as to produce axial loading. The second possibility is that the grinding has removed all contact between the fossa to be restored and the opposing cusp tip.

However, when the occlusal contacts between the inclines are eliminated, so is any occlusal traumatism between the teeth in the MICP. Why? Because horizontal forces and occlusal traumatism result when inclines contact each other. When the *only* contact is between a cusp tip and its opposing fossa, the result is an axial force (Fig. 13C).

IV. Preparation

Prepare the tooth to be restored as usual. Pack the amalgam as usual (Fig. 13D).

V. Gross-Carve the Restoration

Gross-carve the restoration with a *large* discoid instrument; a large discoid is less likely to gouge or overcarve the fossa area. Use of the remaining enamel inclines to guide the discoid will result in an accurate carving. Students often worry about fracturing the proximal box. To eliminate this concern, the matrix band can be trimmed so that the patient can close in the MICP with the matrix in place. In this way the occlusion can be carved prior to removing the matrix. Most experienced dentists do not find trimming the matrix band necessary.

VI. Mark the Restoration

Remove the matrix, if any, and have the patient close gently on the restoration. Let the patient "feel" the new restoration by tapping very, very lightly. (Warn the patient about the possibility of breaking the new restoration.) In this way the opposing cusp tip often makes a mark in the restoration that can be seen in the freshly packed amalgam. If a mark cannot be seen, the teeth are dried and dry articulating ribbon is used. The patient should then be asked to tap his teeth gently on the ribbon. For further insurance with Class II amalgam restorations, it is a good idea to jiggle the patient's jaw and guide the mandible to close lightly on the proximal portion of the restoration.

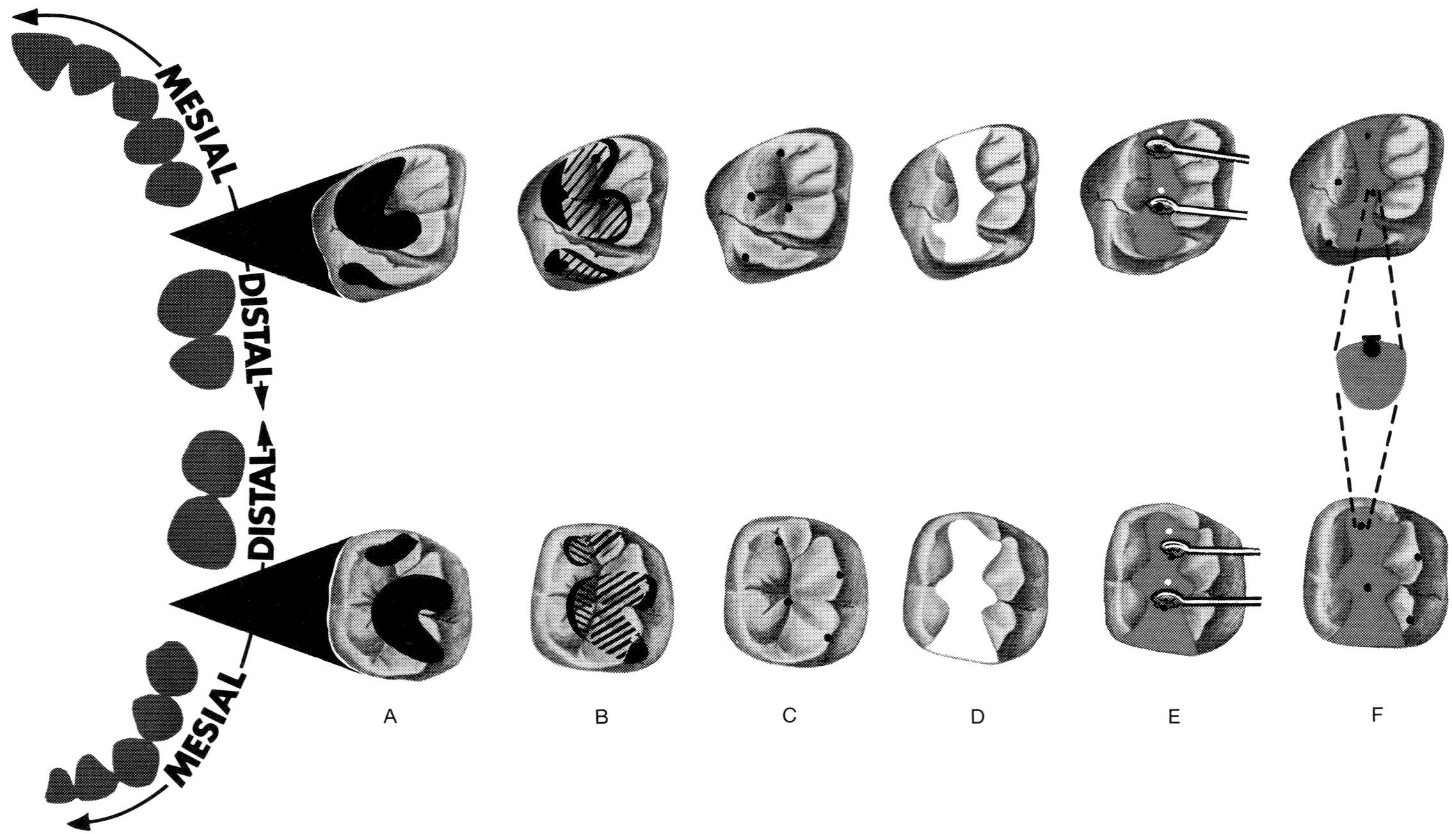

MESIAL
DISTAL
DISTAL
MESIAL
A
B
C
D
E
F

Explain that the restoration is like an egg shell, that it can easily crack.

VII. *Adjust the Occlusion on the Restoration*

Because of the occlusal examination and the occlusal adjustment prior to the preparation of the tooth, it is unlikely that any inclines of the new restoration will contact the opposing tooth. However, if contact marks are noted on the inclines of the new restoration, they should be scraped away, leaving only the contact in the base of the fossa. Then adjust the high restoration with a *large* discoid.

When the restoration is high, the rest of the teeth do not touch. The contact made by the opposing cusp tip must now be adjusted until the patient can again bring his teeth together. We call this adjustment to even contact the "dig-in".

The restoration is adjusted to even contact with the other teeth. On an *upper tooth,* place the discoid on the mark and scrape away the mark by moving the discoid in a *distal* direction. The restoration is marked and adjusted until the contact is as equal as possible in pressure to the marks made on the adjacent teeth (Figs. 13E, 14A). On a *lower tooth,* place the discoid on the mark and scrape away the mark by moving the instrument in a *mesial* direction. Repeat the marking and adjusting of the restora-

FIG. 13. How to adjust occlusion, place restoration, and make cusp seats. Top drawings show upper tooth, bottom drawings lower tooth. **A,** Tooth marked. **B,** Marks on cuspal inclines (*hatched lines*) ground away. Solid black areas represent additional grinding necessary to blend adjustment into surrounding tooth structure. Since teeth are not severely worn, only inner inclines of cusps are ground. Contact on outer incline of lower buccal cusp eliminated by grinding inner incline of upper buccal cusp. Contact on outer incline of upper lingual cusp eliminated by grinding inner incline of lower lingual cusp. **C,** After adjustment, only cusp tips and opposing fossae show marks. There are no marks on inclines. **D,** Tooth prepared for filling. **E,** After gross-carving (restoration still slightly high) and marking of filling, final carving creates cusp seats. To make cusp seat on upper tooth, carve mark and a little distally. To make cusp seat on lower tooth, carve mark and a little mesially. **F,** Finished restoration. There are pinpoint contacts between cusp tips and opposing cusp seats. No inclines contact. The dotted lines lead to an enlargement of a schematic cusp seat. The gray area is the freedom area, the dot is the occlusal contact, and the short, heavy, horizontal line represents the holding boundary.

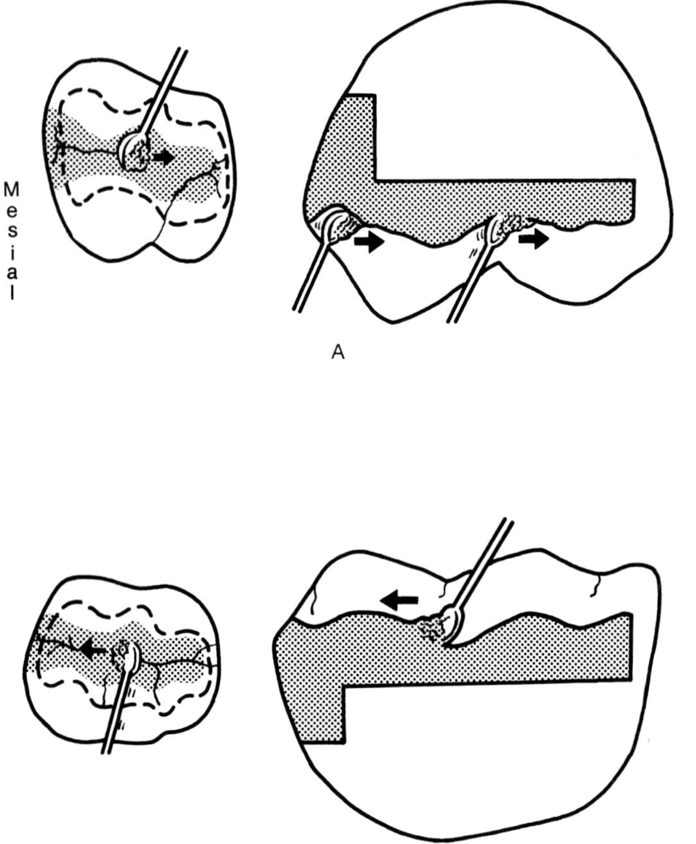

FIG. 14. Dig-in. **A,** On upper tooth, carve dot and a little distally. **B,** On lower tooth, carve dot and a little mesially.

tion until the contact is equal in pressure to the marks of occlusal contact on the adjacent teeth (Figs. 13E, 14B).

This type of carving—dot-and-distal on an upper amalgam (wax, gold, etc.); dot-and-mesial on a lower amalgam (wax, gold, etc.)—automatically creates the occlusal objectives; namely, axial forces, a holding boundary or reference area, and freedom.

If the amalgam has set up too hard to carve with a large discoid, use a large round burr. A #10 or #11 steel burr or a comparable round stone is good. Move the burr in the same way as in scraping with the large discoid.

After the restoration has been adjusted so that it is

hitting evenly with all the other teeth, it is necessary to refine the contact mark to pinpoint size. To do that, retain the deepest pinpoint spot of the mark and lightly grind or scrape the remainder of the mark away.

A common error made by students during the creation of a cusp-seat pinpoint contact is to continue the dig-in technique during the refining procedure. *Do not do* the dot-and-distal on an upper restoration or the dot-and-mesial on a lower restoration once all the teeth in the arch are striking. The dig-in is done *only* when the restoration is *high.* Once the restoration is no longer high, the contact dot is *never* removed; it is refined to pinpoint size (Figs. 13F, 15).

During a dig-in procedure, there is also the option of shortening the supporting cusp tip. This is often done on upper lingual cusps because they do not wear as much as lower buccal cusps (Figs. 61, 79).

In digging-in a long upper lingual cusp, it does not make sense to deepen an already deep fossa area. It would be wiser to shorten the upper lingual cusp tip from mesial to distal. Remember, the distal portion of the upper lingual cusp tip is the holding area of the cusp tip; that is the reason for grinding from mesial to distal.

Next, check the refining process by having the patient "chop, chop" on the ribbon again. The refining procedure may have to be repeated until the mark is tiny.

The result of refining to a pinpoint contact may not be a pinpoint dot, but rather a thin line. This is because we

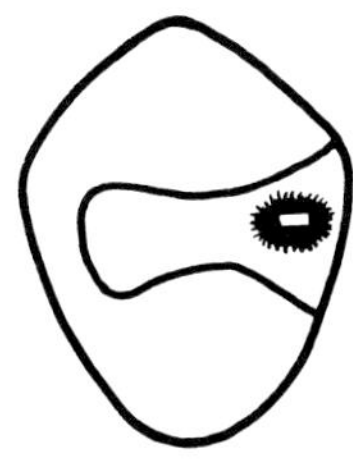
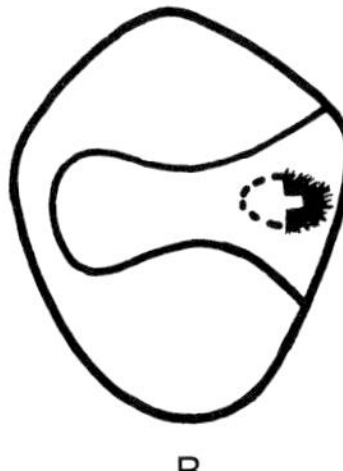
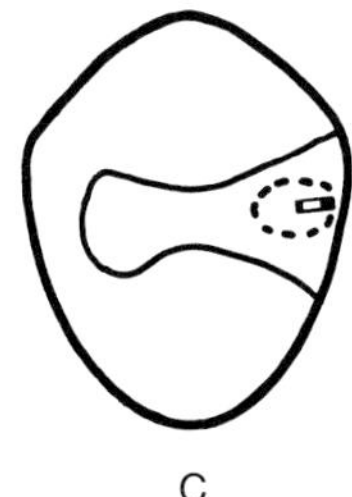
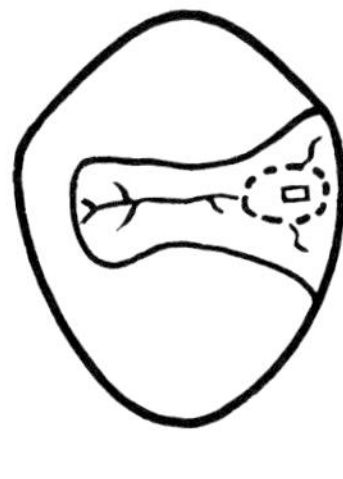

A   B   C   D

FIG. 15. Refining contact dot on upper restoration to pinpoint contact. **A,** Deepest point of mark is noted as white rectangle. **B,** Mark distal to it is scraped away. **C,** Markings buccal and lingual to it are scraped away. **D,** Any mark more than one to two millimeters mesial to deepest pinpoint mark is scraped away.

permit one or two millimeters of contact on the holding boundary. However, the contact must be very thin buccolingually so that there will be complete freedom during lateral motion.

To refine a mark on a lower cusp seat, follow the same technique as with the upper cusp seat, except reverse the mesial and distal.

When adjusting restorations, never use instruments with sharp corners, such as cleoids and square-edged wheels. Use large round burrs or wheels with rounded edges along with the large discoid.

Be sure the mark of contact on the cusp seat is represented by a mark *on* a smooth surface rather than a small gouge *in* the surface of a cusp seat. By adjusting the occlusion on a restoration in this way, a cusp seat is automatically created that results in axial forces on the teeth. The restoration will knock the teeth in instead of out.

By adjusting the mark and distal to it on an upper tooth, and the mark and mesial to it on a lower tooth, the final pinpoint contact will be right on the base of the holding boundary as it joins the freedom area of the cusp seat (Fig. 16). This pinpoint contact will be stable. Remember, the mark from occlusal contact should be pinpoint; it must not be a large mark on the tooth.

Since it is not always possible to get the contact perfect at the first appointment when placing an amalgam, it should be checked in a few days. However, if you follow the adjustment procedure outlined here you will be very accurate.

If any restoration is gouged from contact with an opposing cusp tip because it was left high, it should be adjusted. A large round burr (#10 or #12) should be used. Leave only the deepest pinpoint contact of the gouge mark (Fig. 15).

Occlusal contacts must be pinpoint in size, regardless of the shape of the cusp tip. A pointed cusp, a rounded cusp, or a very broad cusp should still make only a pinpoint contact.

Cusps should not be distorted to achieve pinpoint contact. They may be slightly reshaped, but generally the cusp seats are made to fit the opposing cusp tips (Fig. 17).

Both pinpoint and broad contacts can result in axial

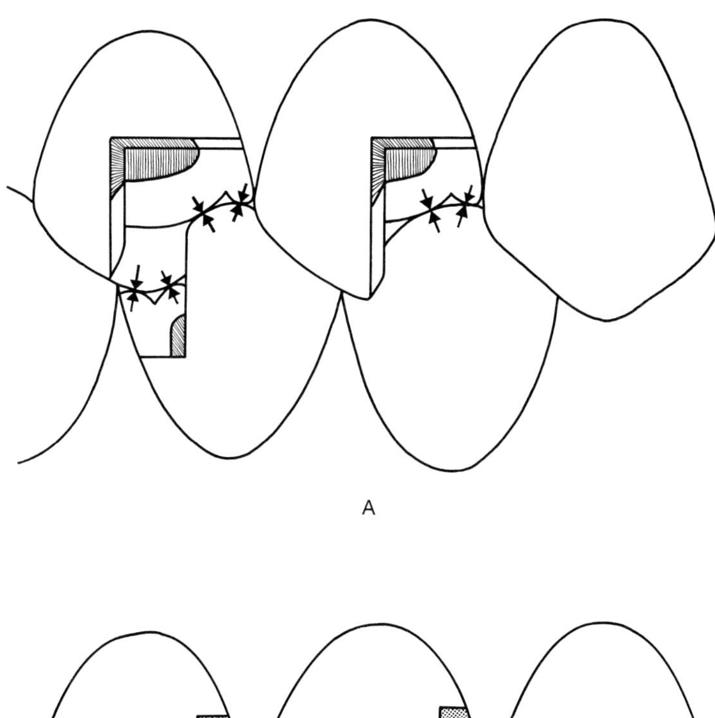

A

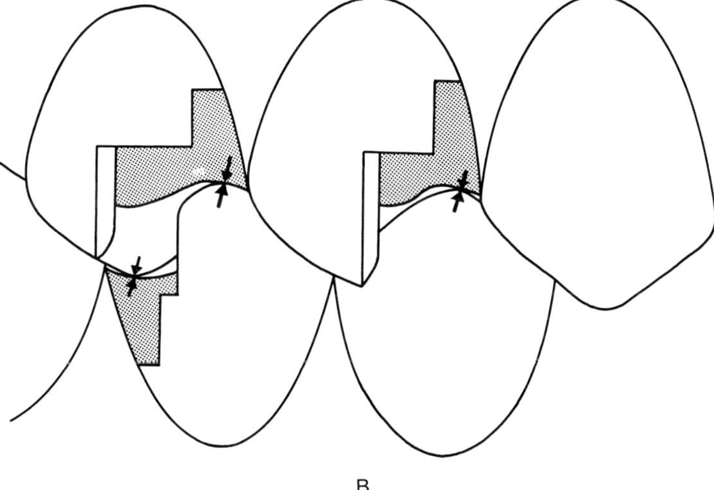

B

FIG. 16. Multiple contacts of carious fossa replaced with single contact of cusp seat. **A,** Cusp tip making multiple contacts in opposing fossa. **B,** Fossa with multiple contacts has been replaced by cusp seat with one pinpoint contact.

forces in a static position. However, the broad large areas of contact can be occlusal interferences for excursive jaw movements. This will become apparent when lateral jaw movement is discussed (pp. 38–40).

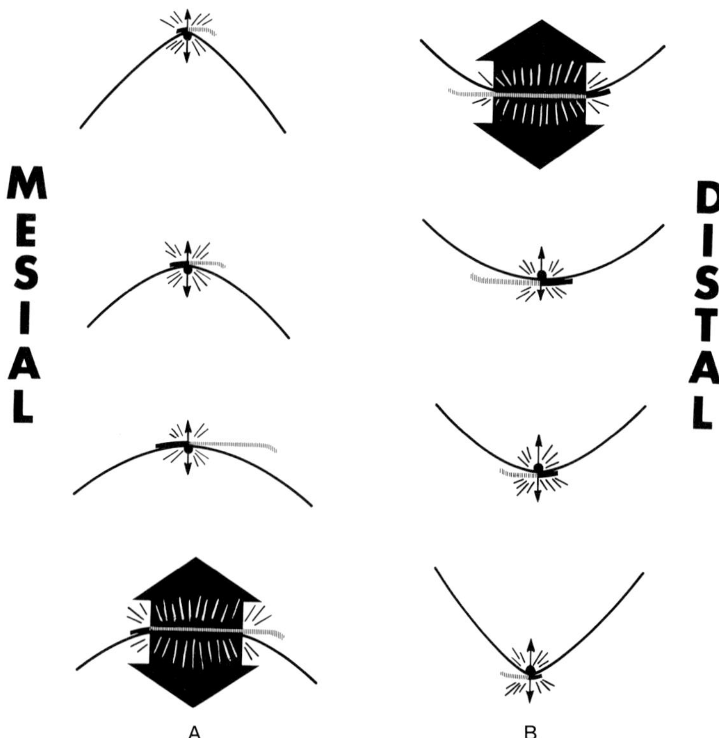

FIG. 17. Regardless of shape of cusp tip, contact can be refined to pinpoint. Drawing shows pointed, rounded, and very broad cusp tips, all refined to pinpoint contacts. Large contact (*heavy arrow*) is incorrect because it would axially load *only* in one static position. Solid line represents holding boundary; striped line represents freedom area. *A,* Lower cusp tip contacting upper tooth. *B,* Upper cusp tip contacting lower tooth.

Once the cusp seat is completed, the contact point should not be touched. All the carving that is customary can be done after the cusp seat has been created. However, do not carve pits or grooves in the cusp seat. Pits and grooves can be placed wherever desirable outside the cusp seat, but no further work should be done in the cusp seat or on the opposing cusp tip.

A POSITIVE AND A STABLE OCCLUSION.   The dig-in procedure establishes a positive occlusion, and it programs the patient to close to this occlusion. Combined with freedom, it results in a stable occlusion. A single point contact provides a positive and stable occlusion. The placement of the contact at the base of the holding boundary positively stabilizes the mandible.

A patient should not have occlusal contacts imposed upon him too much. It is the patient who closes and moves the jaw (and maybe not always precisely the same way), and this fact necessitates simplicity and maximum freedom of occlusion. The cusp seat with one single pinpoint contact achieves these.

Cusp-To-Marginal-Ridge Relationship

A second occlusal relationship encountered while placing restorations occurs when a cusp tip occludes between two marginal ridges (Fig. 18B). This is a simple relationship to restore. The technique requires only minor variations from the technique for the cusp-to-fossa relationship (Fig. 13). Steps I through IV are the same. The only change is in Step V. To adjust the contact from an opposing cusp tip on a marginal ridge, simply

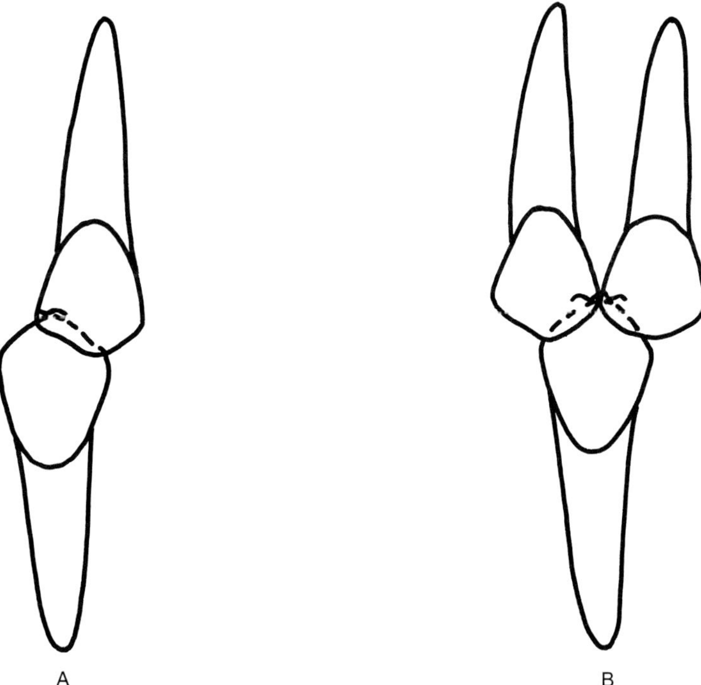

FIG. 18. *A,* Tooth-to-one-tooth occlusion (cusp-to-fossa). Cusp tip occludes within opposing occlusal table. *B,* Tooth-to-two-teeth occlusion (cusp-to-marginal-ridge). Cusp tip is between two marginal ridges.

scrape the marginal-ridge area of the restoration until the pin-point contact is as equal in pressure as possible to the occlusal contacts on adjacent teeth. (Figs. 19, 20). However, a cusp-to-marginal-ridge contact in the occlusion will usually occur on a slight incline of the marginal ridge. (An exception would be in a severely worn dentition.) But since this type of contract can produce slight horizontal forces and wedge the teeth apart, one or both of the following safety factors should be present before placing a restoration with a cusp-to-marginal-ridge relationship.

1.   To offset a marginal-ridge contact and maintain axial forces on the tooth, strong proximal contacts with the teeth mesial and distal to the two teeth involved are needed. Dental floss should meet good resistance when it is placed between these proximal contacts. By stabilizing the teeth, proximal contacts aid in producing axial forces (Fig. 21).

2.   The tooth to be restored should have another occlusal contact that results in axial forces. An example of this would be a molar whose central fossa area provides axial loading on the tooth. In this case a mesial or distal marginal-ridge contact would not wedge or deflect the teeth as long as the two contacts were of equal pressure or in harmony with each other.

If neither of these safety factors is present on the tooth to be filled, then a cusp-to-marginal-ridge relationship should not be restored on this tooth. The opposing cusp tip should be moved mesially or distally to the nearest opposite fossa by means of a crown or onlay. The occlusion can then be treated the same way a cusp-to-fossa relationship is (pp. 16–20).

If one of the safety factors does exist, there is still another problem with the cusp-to-marginal-ridge occlusal relationship. Although usually an insignificant problem, it is included for the sake of completeness. An opposing lower cusp tip may have minor restriction of freedom to move distally from the MICP point of contact to centric relation. In this case it would have to bump into the marginal ridge. An upper opposing cusp tip may also be prevented from taking a more mesial relation to the mandibular tooth if the patient desires to close toward centric relation occlusion or the terminal hinge closure.

If both MICP and centric relation occlusion are the same,

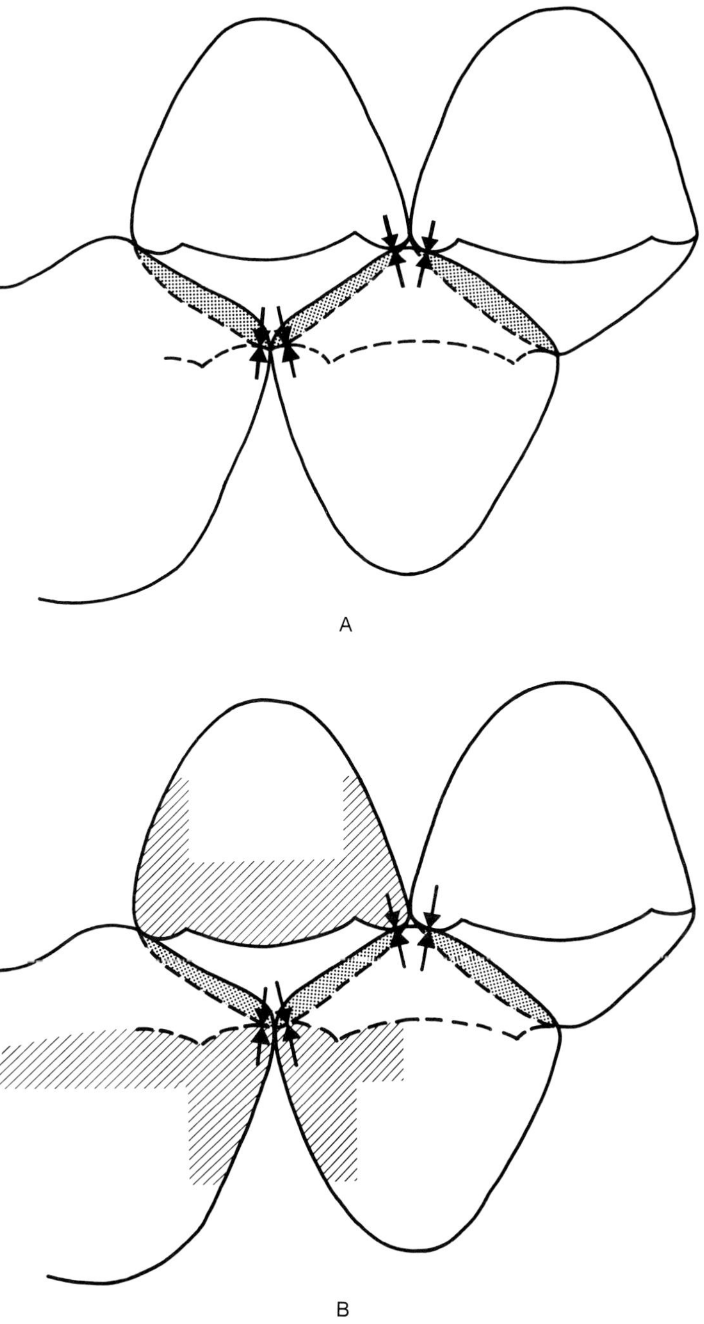

FIG. 19.   Restoring cusp-to-marginal-ridges relationship. **A,** Original cusp-to-marginal-ridges contacts. **B,** Restorations replace cusp-to-marginal ridges contacts. Note that cusp seat has two points of contact in cusp-to-marginal-ridges relationship.

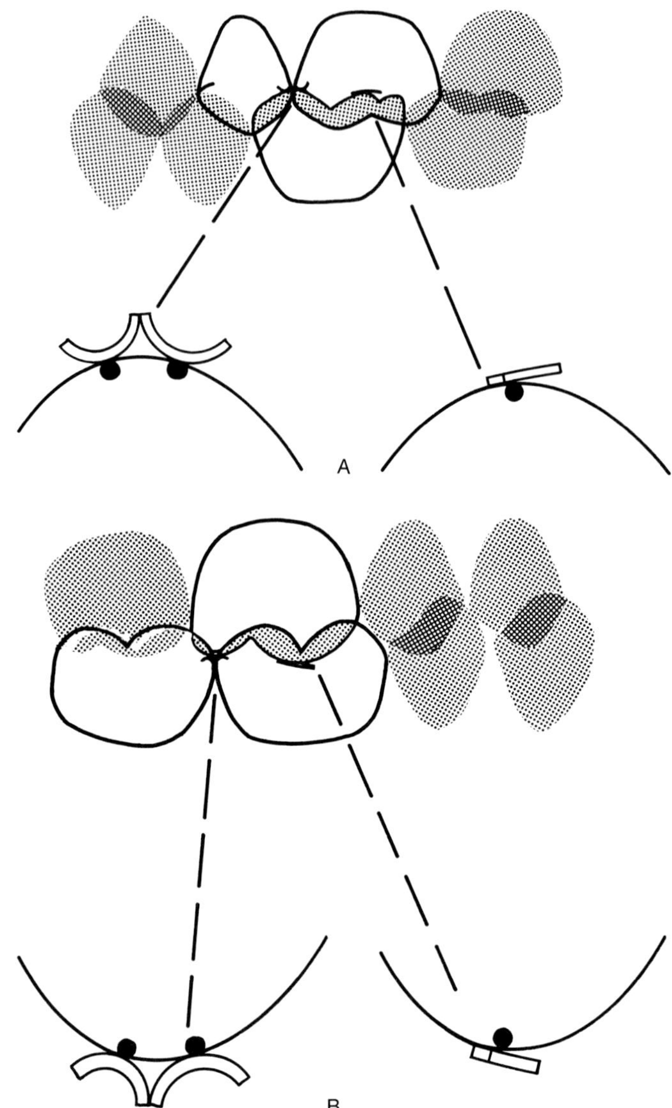

FIG. 20. *A,* Mesiobuccal cusp of lower first molar occludes between two marginal ridges, and middle buccal cusp occludes in central fossa of upper tooth. Cusp-to-fossa relationship has one pinpoint contact with holding boundary mesial to it and has freedom distal to it. Cusp-to-marginal-ridges relationship divides contact into two pinpoint spots of contact, one on each marginal ridge. Contact on most mesial of two contacted marginal ridges acts as holding boundary; contact on more distal of contacted marginal ridges allows freedom posterior to centric relation. *B,* Distolingual cusp of upper first molar occludes between two marginal ridges; mesiolingual cusp occludes in central fossa of lower first molar. Relationships are the same as described in *A,* except that in lower arch holding boundaries are distal to contact points and freedom areas are mesial to contact points.

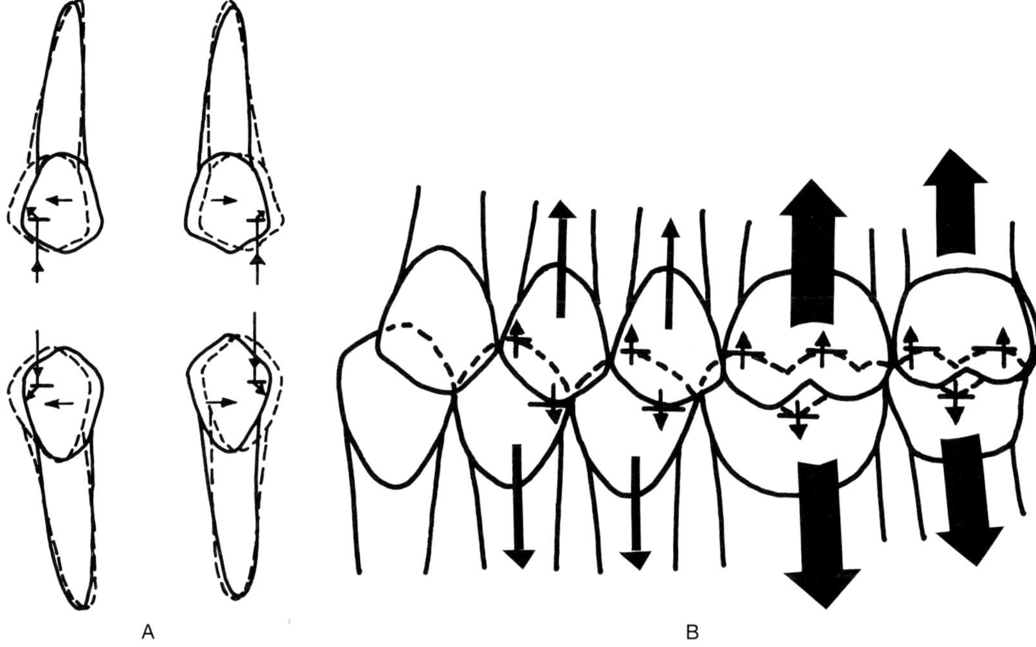

A

B

FIG. 21. *A,* Cusp tips articulating in fossa and marginal-ridge areas without proximal contact can tip teeth. Teeth are not axially loaded unless there are proximal contacts. *B,* Teeth are axially loaded. Proximal contacts prevent tipping of teeth, and occlusal forces are directed axially. Articulation in central fossa of a molar can cause total axial loading of molars, independent of the remainder of the dental arch or of proximal contacts.

there is no problem. If MICP and centric relation occlusion are not the same, the opposing cusp tip may require adjustment to provide freedom to reach centric relation. Freedom for the opposing cusp can be established by flattening the cusp tip between the two points of contact with the marginal ridges. This will allow the mandible to close in centric relation and still axially load the teeth (Fig. 22).

Cusp-To-Incline Relationship

Steps I through IV are the same as those described for the cusp-to-fossa relationship. Overpack the filling material. Gross-carve the material, but leave enough filling material so that a ledge can be made on the cuspal incline. Step V is the same as before. Simply carve a cusp seat on the ledge of filling material (Fig. 23).

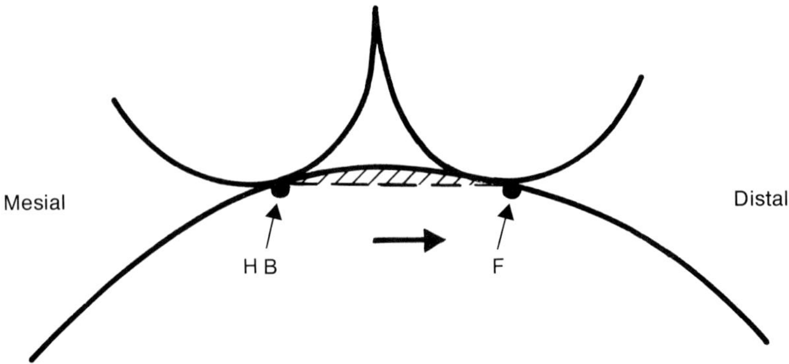

FIG. 22. Cusp tip flattened to allow freedom to centric relation in cusp-to-marginal-ridge relationship. *HB* is the holding boundary contact. *F* is second contact dot, which is free to move distally because there is no incline distal to it. In some situations, in addition to flattening cusp tip, it might be necessary to flatten marginal ridge distal to contact dot. To see what would be done with upper cusp tip, turn drawing upside down and reverse labels *Mesial* and *Distal*.

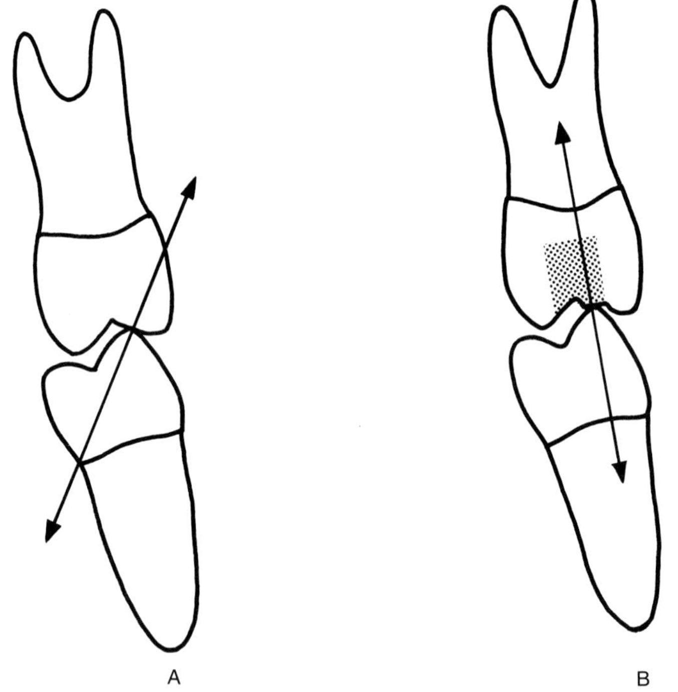

FIG. 23. *A,* Cusp contacting on incline results in horizontal forces. *B,* With a restoration, incline relationship changed to cusp-to-cusp-seat relationship. Forces now more axial.

If the cusp of one tooth strikes on an incline near the tip of another cusp, it may be impossible to create a cusp seat on the tooth by overpacking the filling material. If so, there are three choices:

1. Fill the tooth and leave a light contact on the incline. If the tooth has good proximal contact, it will serve as a space maintainer in the arch. This is an important occlusal function, provided there are enough other teeth in the arch that can be axially loaded for mandibular stability.

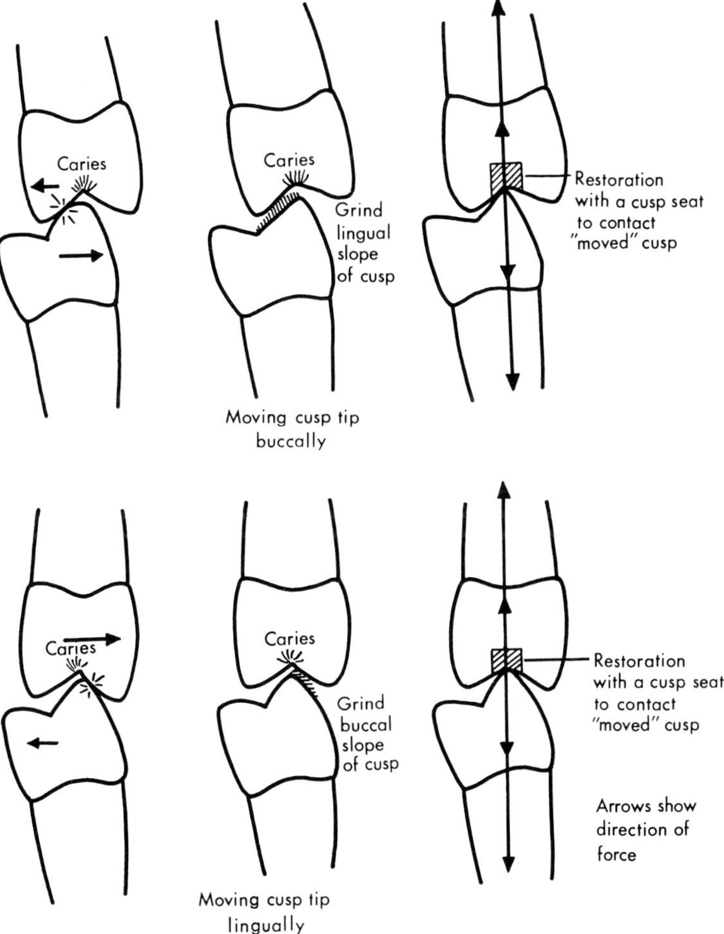

FIG. 24. Cusp tips can be moved opposite fossae prior to restoring teeth. However, grinding shortens cusp. Contact is reestablished with new restorations, or, as discussed on page 32, supporting cusps are shortened.

2. If the tooth must support the occlusion, a crown, onlay, or tooth movement must be used to place a cusp seat opposite a cusp tip for axial loading.

3. When a fossa is to be replaced with a restoration, the cusp opposite the fossa often contacts an incline. This opposing cusp can often be reshaped so that the tip is moved opposite the fossa to be restored (Fig. 24). The reshaping shortens the cusp and takes it out of the contact. However, when the restoration is placed it can be packed so as to reestablish contact with the cusp tip. Often, when only one restoration is being placed, only a primary occlusal contact will be established. The occlusal relationship, although not perfect, will be improved. The tongue, cheek, and proximal contacts will help prevent the teeth from tipping and will help maintain axial loading.

Cusp-To-Cusp Relationship

To axially load the teeth in this situation, slightly flatten the cusps involved (if they are not already flat) and construct an onlay or crown that will occlude with the flattened cusp tip. This will produce the axial force.

To have the onlay or crown also hold or have a holding boundary, simply let the flattened cusp tip incline slightly. It should be inclined superiorly from mesial to distal. In this way the mandible will be kept from slipping mesially and will be held stable (Fig. 25).

Crossbite Relationship

The crossbite is treated as a regular interarch relationship, except that the working cusps are the lower lingual cusps instead of the lower buccal cusps and the upper buccal cusps instead of the upper lingual cusps.

RESTRAINT: THE REASON UPPER MOLARS ARE LOST FIRST

Freedom in the cusp seat—why?

There should be freedom to the distal of the contact point in the upper cusp seat and freedom to the mesial of the contact point in the lower cusp seat.

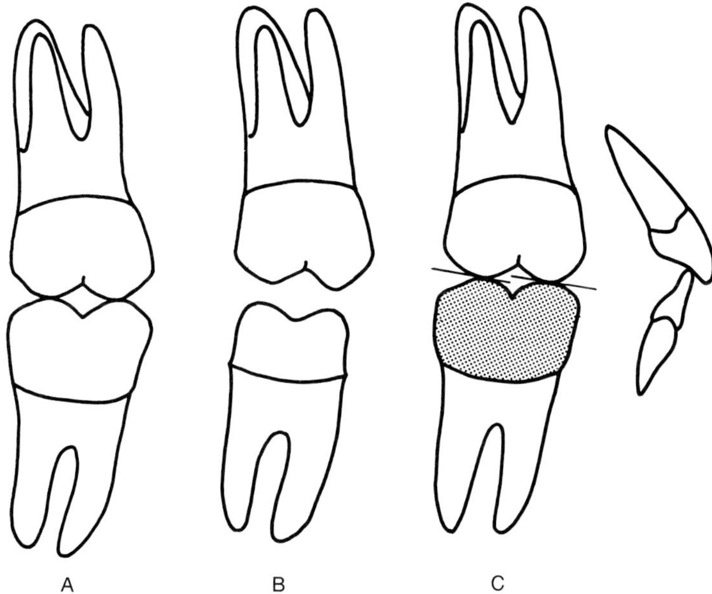

FIG. 25. Changing a cusp-to-cusp relationship without holding boundaries to a cusp-to-cusp-seat relationship with holding boundaries by means of a crown. **A,** Original cusp-to-cusp relationship without holding boundaries. **B,** Lower tooth prepared for crown. **C,** Crown in place has cusp tips flattened and angled slightly so that they now form holding boundaries, and lower tooth and jaw cannot slide mesially with possible trauma to anterior teeth.

According to many studies, most people with a "normal and healthy" dentition have a MICP that is slightly anterior to centric relation. Centric relation will be discussed later. Suffice it to say here that when the mandible goes from an anterior MICP back to centric relation, it moves distally. The lower cusp tips move distally in relation to their upper cusp seats (Fig. 26), and the lower cusp seats move distally in relation to their upper cusp tips (Fig. 27).

If restorations were placed that did not have this freedom, they would have centric restraining inclines immediately next to the point of contact. This would not cause any occlusal trauma so long as the patient always used his anterior MICP. However, under stress, and occasionally during swallowing, people have a tendency to go toward centric relation as well as to the MICP. If there is no restraint to centric relation, there is no harm done. If there is restraint, it may induce bruxing. That is why there must be freedom to the *distal* of the contact point on the upper cusp seat and to the *mesial* of the contact point on the lower cusp seat. With freedom, if the patient should move

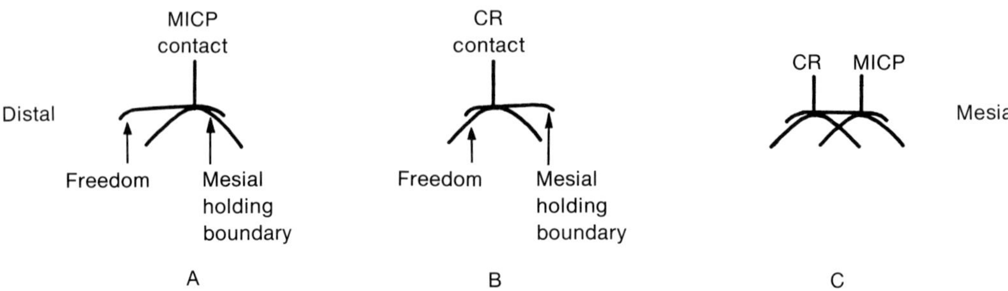

FIG. 26. **A,** Holding boundary programs lower cusp tip to close directly to its base. **B,** There is freedom posteriorly. **C,** Cusp tip, although programed to MICP, is free to close on a flat area anywhere between MICP and CR.

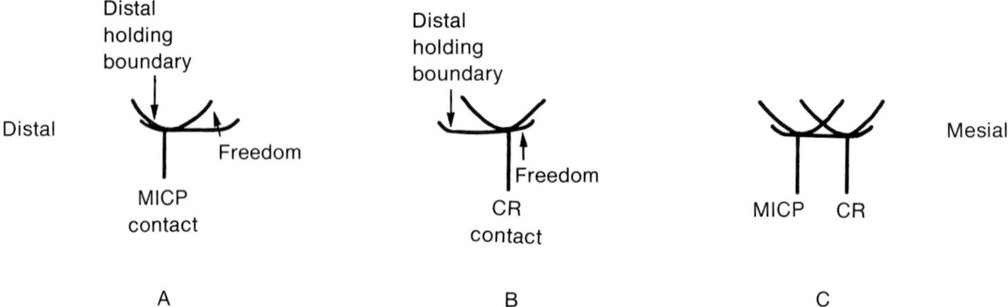

FIG. 27. **A,** Lower cusp seat programed to close to MICP. **B,** Lower cusp seat has freedom mesial to contact point. **C,** Upper cusp tip can be hit anywhere between MICP and CR and be on a flat plane.

his jaw distally from an anterior MICP, the cusp tips would move onto this flattened area and thus maintain axial loading.

A restoration placed in the MICP without freedom to centric relation can cause occlusal traumatism and open the contact between the last upper molars (Fig. 28).

Placing restorations with the cusp-seat anatomy will insure axial loading of the teeth no matter which path of closure the patient uses. The teeth will not be deflected, there will be no occlusal traumatism, and contacts will remain closed.

Practically speaking, a dentist cannot adjust every patient's occlusion so that the MICP is the same as centric relation. It cannot even be said that this would be desirable if it were practical. Neither can every dentist mount every case on a fully adjustable articular and trace out the exact mandibular movements so that each restoration can be carved to fit perfectly the

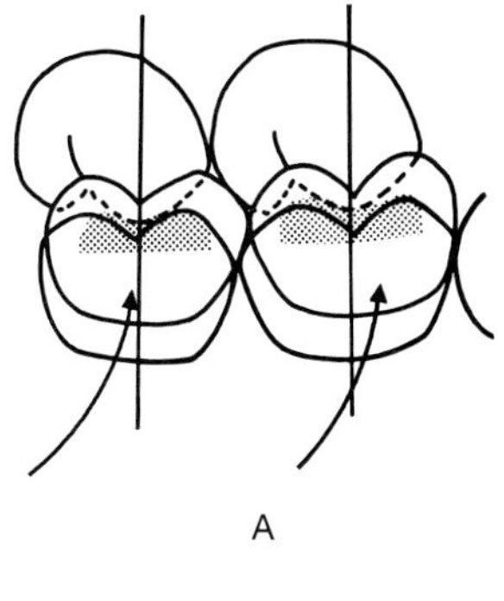

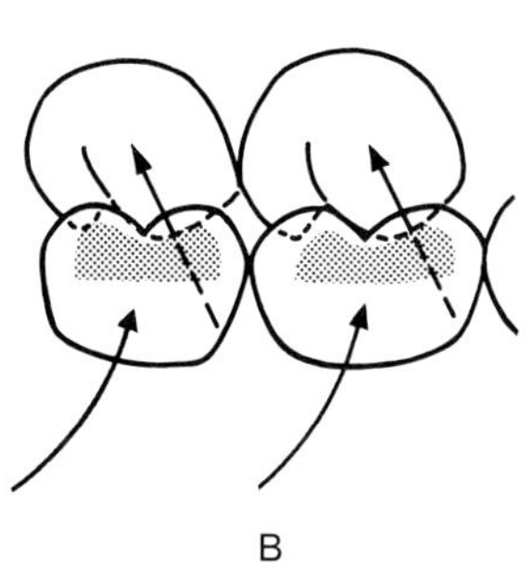

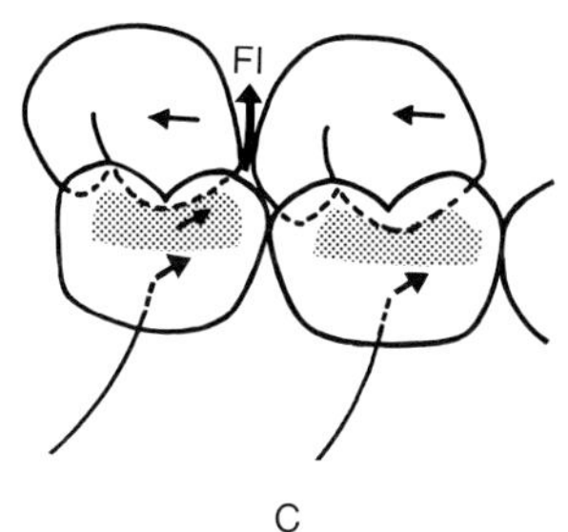

patient's every mandibular movement. What can be done is to use cusp seats to support the teeth with an axial load. The cusp seat will automatically provide the necessary freedom so that the mandible can be stabilized in the MICP and not restrained from centric relation. The teeth will be pushed into their sockets whenever the patient closes. There will be no restraint, and bruxing will not be encouraged.

Naturally, the single restoration by itself cannot provide freedom for mandibular movements when the rest of the teeth are unchanged. The remainder of the teeth will be discussed later. The technique described here occludes correctly at least a couple of teeth.

FIG. 28. Occlusal restoration on a lower second molar. **A,** Filling in lower tooth has no freedom to centric relation. All force is axial as long as mandible closes on direct arc to MICP. **B,** When mandible closes into centric relation, the disto-occlusal incline on the restoration strikes the upper lingual cusp prematurely, initiating distal force on upper molars. **C,** Lower teeth then slide on inclines mesially and occlusally, pushing upper molars distally, opening their contacts and paving way for food impaction (*FI*) and periodontal destruction.

FOR SELF-EVALUATION

1. What is a cusp seat?

2. What are the three parts of a cusp seat?

3. Which of these parts insures that the restoration does not allow the mandible to slip forward?

4. Which of these parts insures that the restoration does not restrain any mandibular movement?

5. There are both primary and stabilizing contacts between teeth. Which contact best axially loads the teeth?

6. In normally related teeth, the primary occlusal contact occurs between the ______________ _______________ ______________ _______________ and their opposing fossae or marginal ridges.

7. What is the proper contact between cuspal inclines?

3

Providing Lateral Freedom
(*The Lateral Index*)

Excursive movements of the mandible should be unrestrained, without interference. This has long been an objective of occlusal treatment. To achieve this objective we use the concept of the lateral pathway. It describes the space through which cusp tips pass during lateral movements once interference has been removed.

The lateral pathway implies both no lateral contact between teeth and freedom of access to and from the MICP. Remember that ideal occlusion means contact of the teeth that produces axial forces on them. If teeth contact during lateral motion, the forces on the teeth will not be perfectly axial. Therefore, *a therapeutic objective in dentistry is to make it unlikely that teeth touch one another during jaw movements.*

How is this objective possible? First, achieving it requires a subtle change in our thinking. Dentists think about how to make teeth contact in excursive jaw movements rather than about how to have the teeth not contact. Numerous occlusal philosophies and instruments are used successfully. But success results not from the particular excursive tooth contacts but rather from the lack of tooth contact. In other words, success occurs when the patients do not use the excursive tooth contacts designed. Whatever the scheme, philosophy, or instrument used, if the teeth do not touch one another during excursive movements, health results. So think how to make the teeth *not* touch in excursive motions.

To do this, you must understand mandibular movement and the various angles of that movement in relation to different teeth. Since the lower teeth move, you must know the direction and angle of their movement and you must relate factors to the upper teeth.

LATERAL MOVEMENT

Lateral movement of the mandible is primarily lateral, with a slight tipping component and a protrusive component (Fig. 29). In this movement, the dentition is divided into a working side and a nonworking side. The working side, or half, of the dentition is the side on which the mandible is functioning. When

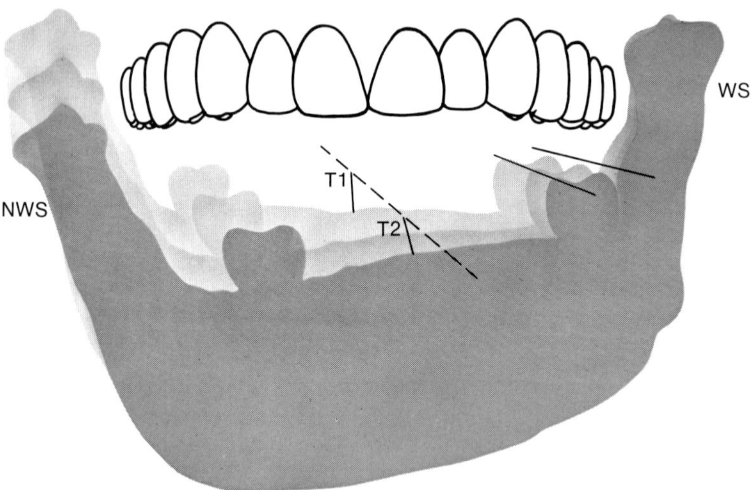

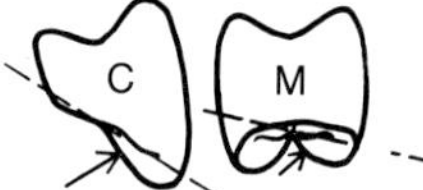

FIG. 29. Lateral mandibular movement related to tooth movement. Tooth on nonworking side (*NWS*) moves more protrusively and downward compared to tooth on working side (*WS*). Tooth on WS moves more laterally and less downward than tooth on NWS. All lower teeth tip during lateral movement because mandible tips (*T1, T2*). Lower buccal cusp of tooth on WS moves at smaller angle than does lingual cusp of same tooth, compared to horizon. Two isolated teeth at left illustrate difference in marginal ridges between cuspid (*C*) and second bicuspid or molar (*M*). Two broken lines indicate relative paths of movement of opposing lower cusp tips during lateral movement. Lateral movement of lower cusp tip tends to follow direction of marginal ridge area of opposing upper tooth. If, instead of marginal-ridge area, the steeper area of cuspal incline (*arrows*) was contacted during lateral movement, contact would be, at least potentially, an occlusal interference. The reason is that contact restrains musculature from moving mandible laterally to same extent and at same angle as marginal ridge area.

one chews on the left side, the left side is the working side and the right side is the nonworking side. Conversely, When one chews on the right side, the right side is the working side and the left side is the nonworking side.

The angles at which the various lower teeth move are related to the horizon or horizontal plane when the head is erect. The angle of motion of the lower teeth becomes smaller as one proceeds around the dental arch from the most distal tooth on the nonworking side to the most distal tooth on the working side. This simple understanding of the lateral jaw movement of the lower teeth will guide you in adjusting a bite to create a lateral pathway (Figs. 30, 31). Since most restorations and occlu-

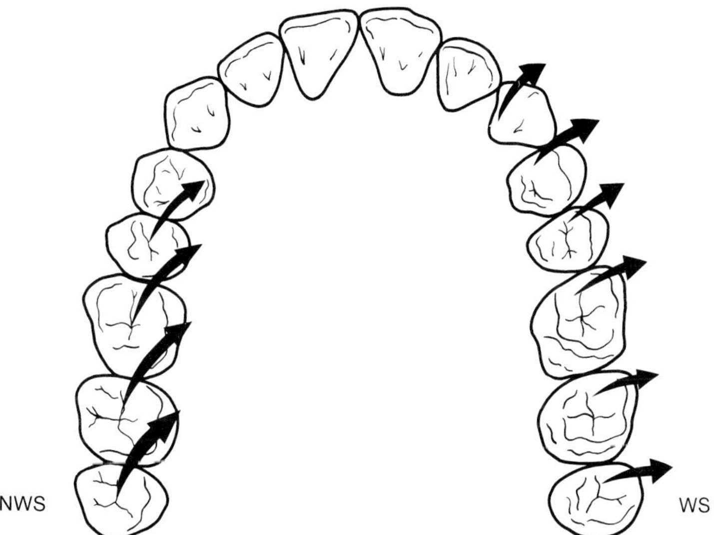

FIG. 30. Arrows indicate movement of lower cusps during lateral jaw movement. Drawing shows lateral movement in horizontal plane, but shape of arrows attempts to show that lower cusps also open. Right half of illustration represents working side (*WS*). Left half represents nonworking side (*NWS*). An important point is that movement on NWS is more protrusive and has more opening than movement on WS. Conversely, WS movement is less protrusive and has less opening. For example, arrow of movement on NWS third molar points more protrusively than arrow on WS third molar. Arrow of NWS movement is larger, indicating more opening of teeth on NWS. Arrow of movement on WS indicates more direct lateral movement with very little opening component. Lateral movement tends to follow natural anatomic grooves in teeth if teeth are in perfect relationship to each other. Since perfect relationship is rarely seen, occlusions need to be adjusted.

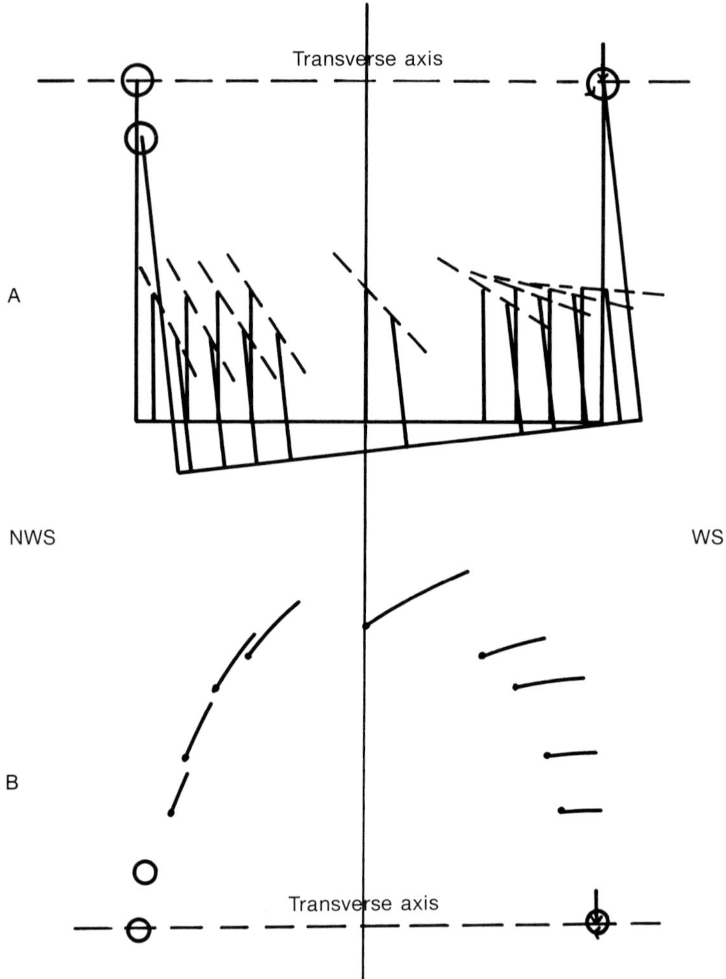

Fig. 31. Schematic representation of lateral jaw movement. *A,* Frontal view. Dashed lines show paths of tooth movement. Circle with arrow shows that working side (*WS*) condyle rotates. Vertical arrow points to sagittal axis. Two circles on nonworking side (*NWS*) show that NWS condyle moves downward and forward. As a result, teeth on WS move more horizontally, while teeth on NWS have a larger vertical component to their lateral movement. *B,* Occlusal view. Circle with arrow shows that WS condyle remains in place and rotates. Vertical arrow points to vertical axis. Condyle on NWS moves forward and medially. As a result, teeth on WS move more directly laterally, while teeth on NWS have larger protrusive component to their lateral movement.

sal adjustments are done directly in the mouth, without the aid of an articulator, this understanding of lateral movement related to the teeth is necessary.

The occlusal objective during excursive jaw movements is no occlusion. But something has to touch somewhere—or does it? No occlusion means that during natural, functional jaw movements there should be no contacting of the cuspal inclines. Natural jaw movements will then be controlled by the neuromuscular mechanism, as it should be. The person concerned will be primarily a chewer rather than a bruxer.

Contact of any cuspal inclines during a jaw movement obstructs and restrains that movement. Interfering with or restraining jaw movement upsets the neuromuscular system and causes bruxism, which, in turn, causes occlusal traumatism (Fig. 32B).

With freedom, the patient opens his mouth, grasps food, and crushes food between the teeth on the movement back to the MICP. The movement will be repeated again and again until the food is chewed and swallowed. During the chewing cycle the teeth hardly touch, and there is no trauma. Traumatism occurs when inclines are placed in the way of the individual's range of

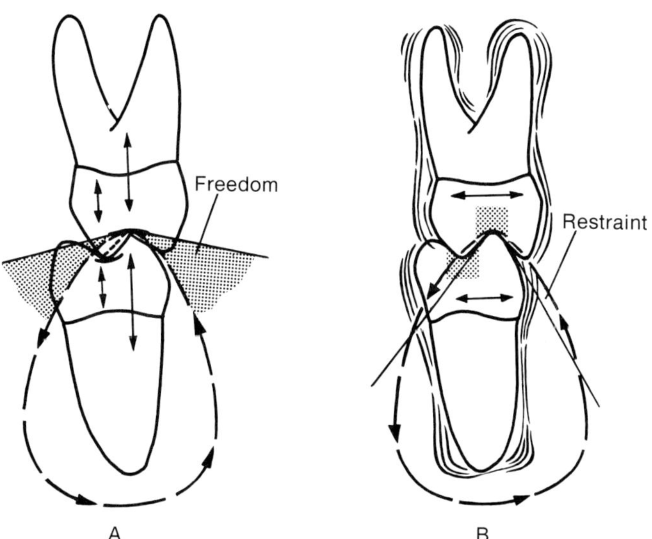

FIG. 32. **A,** Freedom area (*dotted area*) allows for normal and customary range of lateral movement (*curved arrows*) because cusps pass between each other. Arrows on teeth show that force is primarily vertical. **B,** Restraint develops if cusps cannot pass between each other because of malalignment of teeth or because overcarved restorations allowed teeth to erupt more deeply into each other. Here cuspal inclines fall within boundary of normal and customary jaw movement (*curved arrows*) and become interferences. Lines of motion around teeth indicate that luxation now takes place. Arrows on teeth indicate that force is primarily horizontal.

jaw motion, often inducing bruxism. An example is a case in which a cusp tip contacts in the middle of a bicuspid (Fig. 33).

Since tooth contact is possible during lateral movement it is the dentist's responsibility to insure both maximum freedom of motion without tooth contact and that when contact does occur, it is on as horizontal a tooth surface as possible. This design of a lateral pathway makes tooth contact improbable during lateral movement.

In summary, if any area of a posterior tooth contacts, other than the very tips of supporting cusps, bases of fossae, marginal-ridge areas, and grooves, an occlusal interference is likely.

CREATING A LATERAL PATHWAY

When adjusting the occlusion in any excursive motion, it is important not to destroy the MICP contacts.

The creation of the lateral pathway involves the systematic removal of lateral interferences. The first interference to eliminate is the nonworking-side interference.

Elimination of the Nonworking-Side Interference (NWI)

The nonworking side of the dentition is the side opposite the direction of a lateral movement. If the mandible moves to the left, the right side is the nonworking side. If the mandible moves to the right, the left side is the nonworking side. During a lateral movement the nonworking side should not make any occlusal contacts. The instant the patient begins a lateral movement, the teeth on the nonworking side should separate. The only thing the teeth contact on the nonworking side is air.

HOW TO EXAMINE THE NONWORKING SIDE. To examine a tooth or teeth for nonworking-side contact, have the patient make a

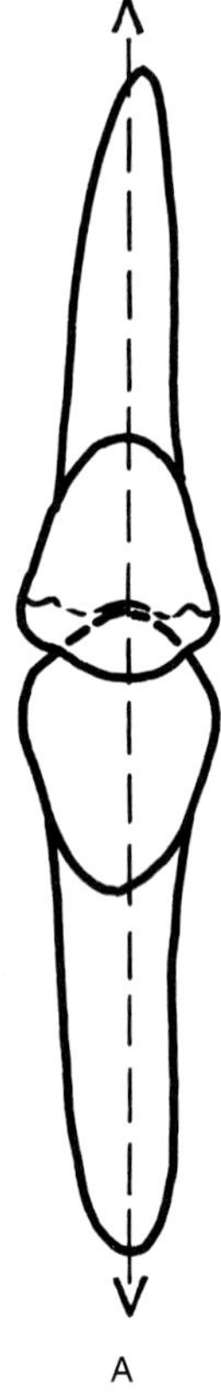

A

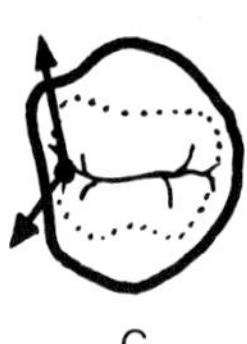

B

C

FIG. 33. Occlusal-relationship problem. *A,* Supporting cusp articulates in middle of opposing tooth, which, although it may produce axial force in MICP, presents a problem during excursive motion. *B,* Occlusal view of *A,* showing lines of motion luxating tooth because cuspal inclines interfere during lateral movement. This problem is manageable by occlusal adjustment in most instances. *C,* Occlusal view, showing no restraint of lateral movement (WS and NWS) when cusps articulate in fossae.

lateral movement toward the opposite side. Guide the patient by pointing with your finger in the direction you want him to move his mandible (Fig. 34). Another method is to place the tip of your index finger on the upper bicuspids on the side toward which you want the patient to move his mandible. Your finger-tip should be on the outer tips of the bicuspid buccal cusps so that it extends below the occlusal plane. Then tell the patient to move his chin sideward until his lower teeth bump or push your finger (Fig. 34).

Merely telling the patient to move his mandible to the left or right can be confusing. Often the patient thinks he is doing exactly what he has been told, while in fact he may not be moving the jaw at all; or he may be moving it in the direction opposite to that desired. When the patient accomplishes the desired movement, praise him: "That's good," "You're doing fine." Be an appreciative doctor and your patients will be more cooperative.

TECHNIQUE

    I.   Place about 3/4 of an inch of articulating ribbon in a hemostat. The ribbon should not extend beyond the tips of the hemostat beaks. One cut edge of the ribbon should be even with one side of the beaks of the hemostat (Fig. 35A).

   II.   Dry the teeth to be checked for nonworking-side contact. Two-inch-square gauze sponges are good for this purpose.

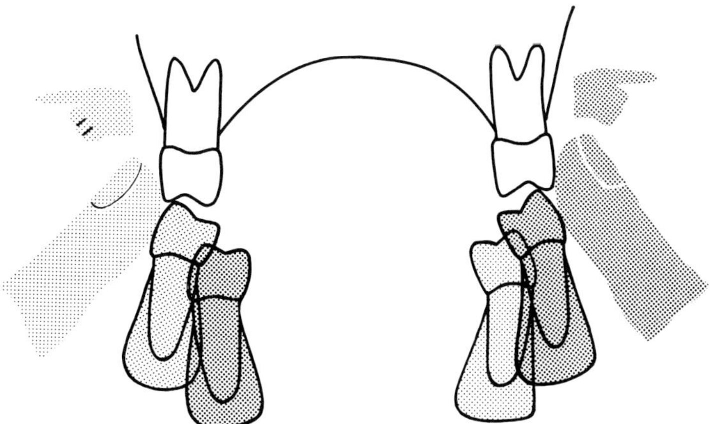

FIG. 34. Help patient to make lateral movement by pointing with finger or by holding finger on side toward which you want patient to move mandible.

III. Place the articulating ribbon between the teeth to be checked and have the patient close in the MICP.

IV. With slight tension, pull laterally on the articulating ribbon with the hemostat. The MICP contact holds the ribbon in place (Fig. 35B).

V. Have the patient move his jaw laterally toward the opposite side. Follow the previously mentioned suggestions for helping the patient make lateral movement (p. 43).

VI. If the ribbon is released the instant the patient moves laterally to the opposite side and remains released throughout the movement, there are no nonworking-side occlusal contacts (interferences). No adjustment of nonworking-side contacts is necessary (Fig. 35C).

VII. If, when pulled gently with the hemostat, the ribbon is not instantly released (Fig. 35D), maintain tension on the ribbon and have the patient continue the lateral movement to the other side until it is released.

VIII. Ask the patient to open as soon as the ribbon is released and to hold his mouth open so as to not erase any marks by wetting the teeth while swallowing. The areas of nonworking-side contact will have been marked by the ribbon.

IX. Grind away the nonworking-side contacts (Fig. 36). Repeat the procedure until ribbon is released the instant lateral movement begins toward the opposite side. Make sure also that the teeth remain out of contact throughout the range of nonworking-side motion (Fig. 35E). (Check each pair of opposing teeth on the nonworking side.)

Sometimes the ribbon on the nonworking side will release the instant a lateral movement begins but will make contact as the movement continues. Make sure that

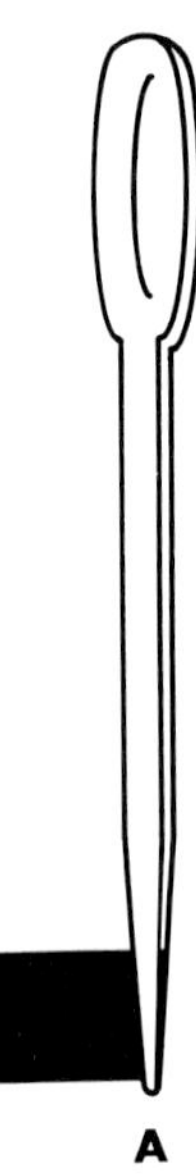

A

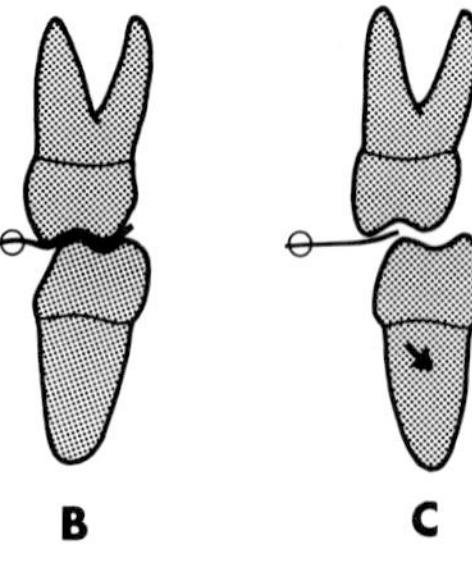

B   C

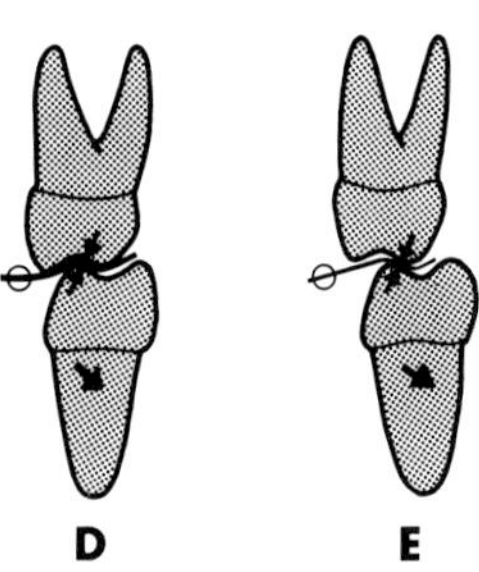

D   E

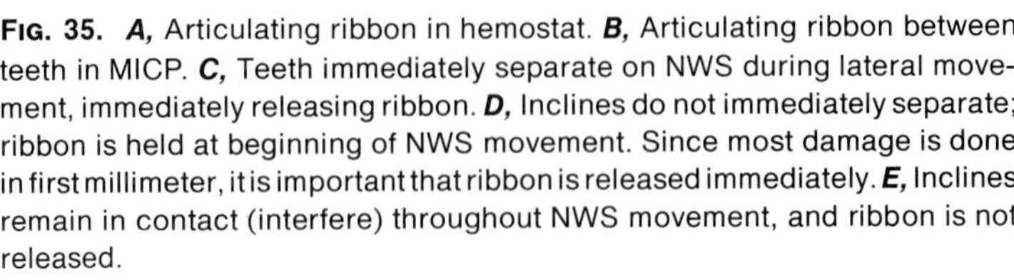

FIG. 35. *A,* Articulating ribbon in hemostat. *B,* Articulating ribbon between teeth in MICP. *C,* Teeth immediately separate on NWS during lateral movement, immediately releasing ribbon. *D,* Inclines do not immediately separate; ribbon is held at beginning of NWS movement. Since most damage is done in first millimeter, it is important that ribbon is released immediately. *E,* Inclines remain in contact (interfere) throughout NWS movement, and ribbon is not released.

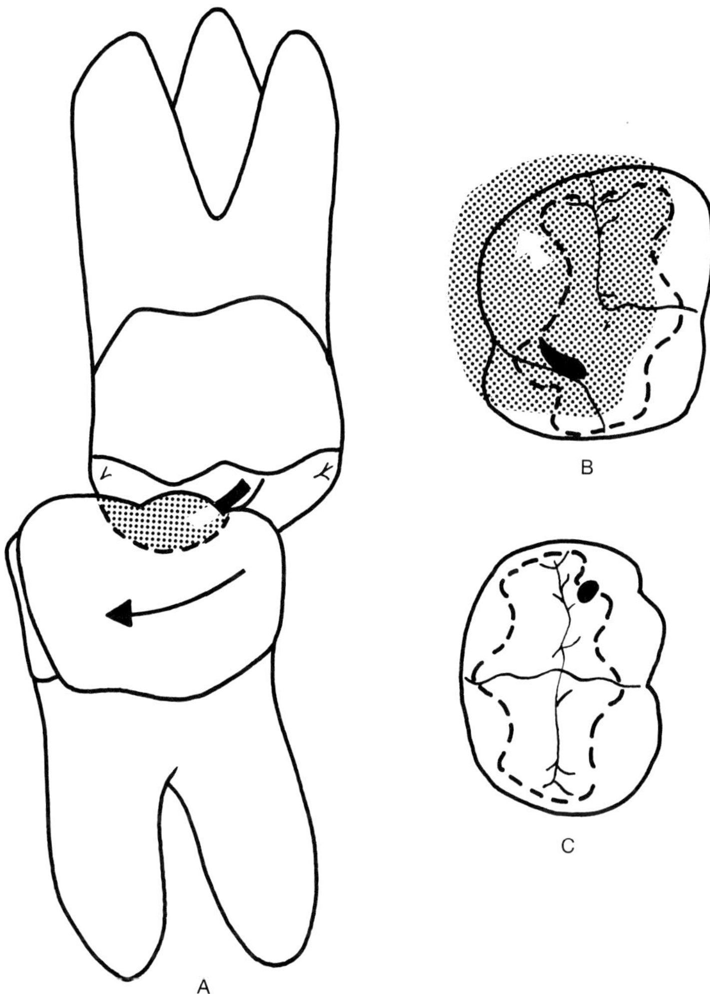

Fɪɢ. 36. **A,** Nonworking-side movement of lower tooth in relation to upper tooth during lateral movement. Lower tooth makes nonworking-side mark on upper tooth during lateral movement. Mark on upper tooth shown by white and black line. **B,** Lower tooth (*shaded*) in relation to upper tooth during nonworking-side movement. Arrow indicates direction in which lower tooth is moving. Nonworking-side interference shown by solid line. **C,** Mark on lower tooth is often smaller than mark on upper tooth. Since lower tooth moves, lower tooth marks upper tooth, just as a pencil makes a line.

there is no occlusal contact on the nonworking side throughout the range of lateral motion.

LOCATION OF THE NONWORKING-SIDE INTERFERENCE. The nonworking-side condyle moves downward, forward, and medially

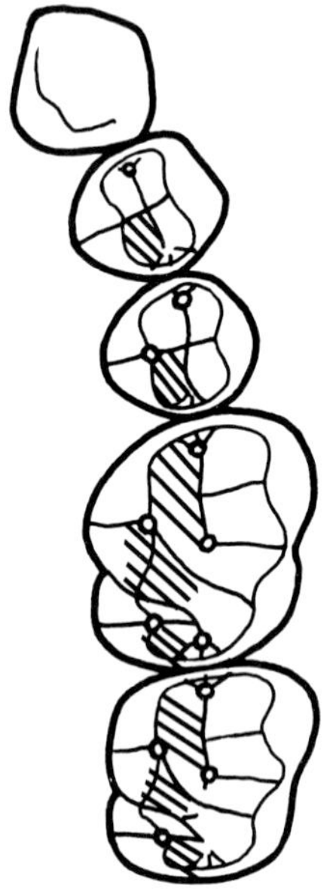

along the articular eminence. The mandibular teeth on the nonworking side, of course, move along with the mandible, downward, forward, and medially. The nonworking-side contact on an upper tooth will thus be on a distal inner incline of the lingual cusp. The nonworking-side contact on a lower tooth will be on a mesial inner incline of the lower buccal cusp (Fig. 37). Except in a crossbite occlusion, the nonworking-side interferences will occur between upper lingual cusps and lower buccal cusps. On malposed or worn teeth, the nonworking-side contacts could occur on and near the cusp tips. The nonworking-side contact, while it can occur anywhere on the nonworking side, will most often be in the molar area.

WHERE AND HOW TO GRIND THE NONWORKING-SIDE INTERFERENCE

Avoid Grinding MICP Contacts out of Occlusion During Correction of Nonworking-Side Interferences

Before grinding nonworking-side interferences, be certain *not* to grind away MICP contacts. (If they are ground away, the teeth will shift because of no occlusion in the MICP.) The only time a MICP contact would be removed is when it is to be replaced immediately with a restoration or when there are other MICP contacts on the same tooth to maintain occlusion.

Distinguish MICP Contacts from Nonworking-Side Interferences

In the examination for nonworking-side contacts, articulating ribbon is used to mark both the MICP contacts and the nonworking-side interferences. The deepest pinpoint spot of the mark in a fossa, marginal ridge, or groove is a MICP mark, as is the pinpoint part of a mark on the *tip* of a supporting cusp. Any other marks are nonworking-side interferences and should be ground away (Fig. 38).

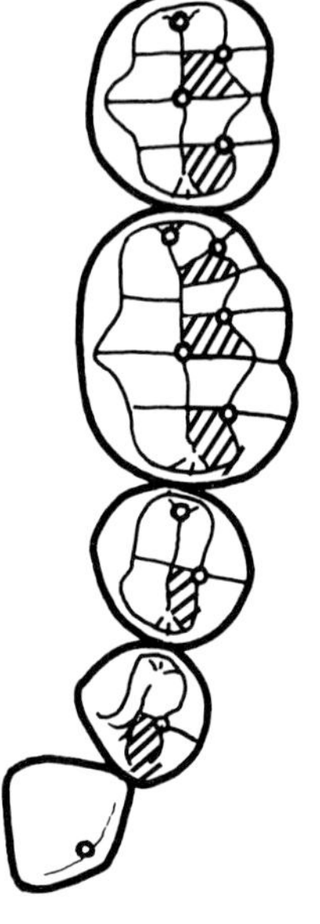

Fig. 37. Small, white circles represent ideal MICP contacts. Oblique lines represent inclines where nonworking-side interferences commonly occur. They are distal inner inclines of upper lingual cusps and mesial inner inclines of lower buccal cusps.

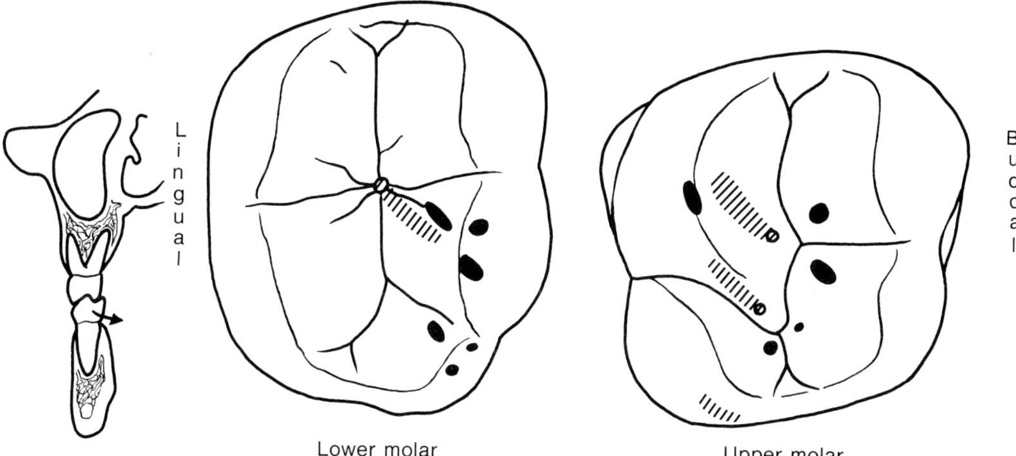

FIG. 38. Streaks of nonworking-side contacts on inner inclines of supporting cusps must be differentiated from MICP contacts that may participate in making these marks. Hatched streak on lower tooth represents mark made by tip of upper lingual cusp during nonworking-side movement. Hatched streaks on upper tooth represent contacts of lower supporting (buccal) cusp tips during nonworking-side movement. Notice that the very tips of lower supporting cusps do not contact in MICP. They are suspended or tripoded in opposing upper fossae. Only mark on inner incline of lower tripoded supporting cusp participates in making or contacting opposing upper tooth during nonworking-side movement. Hatched areas are ground. Circled areas of hatched streaks are MICP contacts of supporting cusps. These circled areas are *not* ground.

Do Most Grinding to Correct Nonworking-Side Interferences on the Upper Tooth

Since the lower buccal cusp occluding in the upper fossa is usually the primary MICP contact for axial loading, it is necessary to maintain as much of this cusp as possible. Nonworking-side contact involves the tip of the lower buccal cusp more often than it does the tip of the upper lingual cusp because of the movement of the lower buccal cusp in the nonworking-side movement. The lower buccal cusp is used in the MICP contact, whereas the distal incline of the upper lingual cusp can easily be sacrificed.

Under certain circumstances, the lower tooth may also be ground. For instance, if the nonworking-side interference is between the inner *incline* of the lower buccal cusp and the *tip* of the upper lingual cusp, the correct procedure is to relieve the lower incline since the upper lingual cusp tip is in a MICP contact.

What should be done if the nonworking-side interference includes both the tip of a lower buccal cusp and the tip of an upper lingual cusp? If both the upper lingual cusp tip and lower buccal cusp tip are contacting in the MICP, the MICP contact on the upper lingual cusp would usually be ground, because it is not the primary occlusal contact for axial loading.

Sometimes a Restoration is Needed

There are instances during a nonworking-side movement when the middle of a lower buccal cusp runs directly into the middle of an upper lingual cusp. It is impossible to grind enough off the upper lingual cusp tip to eliminate the interference without endangering the pulp of the tooth. In this case it is necessary to grind the lower buccal cusp tip until the interference is removed. This results in complete loss of contact between the two teeth. To prevent shifting of the teeth, an upper restoration is needed. The restoration should be made with a cusp seat that contacts the shortened lower buccal cusp in the MICP (Fig. 39).

Determining How Much to Grind

Do you just polish away the ribbon mark, or do you lean on the grinding wheel? The obvious answer is, it all depends. Does the working side contact? If it does, then not much grinding is necessary. Dry the teeth and hold the articulating ribbon between the teeth on both the nonworking and working sides. Have the patient move his jaw laterally toward the working side. Examine the marks on the teeth. Does the mark representing the nonworking-side contact appear lighter, heavier, or the same as the marks representing the lateral contact on the working side?

If the nonworking-side mark is lighter than the working side mark, very little grinding is necessary. Check the results. Be careful of extremely faint marks from articulating ribbon. The teeth may not be contacting. A faint mark can appear due to the thickness of the ribbon. When in doubt, place some cellophane in the hemostat and check for *instant* release of the cellophane when a lateral movement toward the opposite side begins. If the nonworking-side marks are the same as the working-side marks, very little grinding is necessary. If the nonworking-side marks

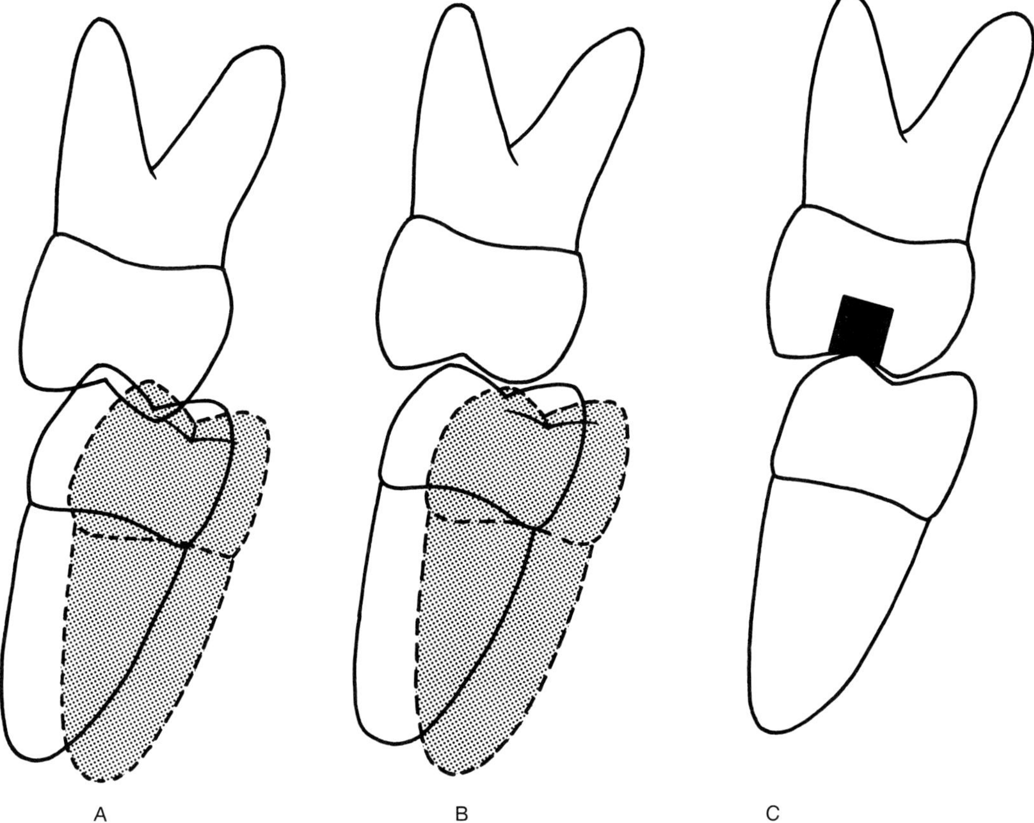

Fig. 39. *A,* Nonworking-side interference. *B,* Upper lingual cusp and lower buccal cusp had to be ground extensively to eliminate nonworking-side interference, resulting in loss of MICP contact. *C,* MICP contact reestablished with restoration in upper tooth.

are heavier than the working-side marks, moderate grinding is necessary. If the nonworking-side interference causes separation of the teeth on the working side during a lateral movement, considerable grinding is necessary.

The amount of grinding needed to eliminate a nonworking-side interference is a matter of judgment. Judgment improves with experience. Do not forget to polish all areas that were ground.

There are some nonworking-side interferences that widely disarticulate the working side. In unusual circumstances of malposed teeth, it may be impossible to eliminate the nonworking-side interference without danger to the pulps of the teeth. These situations may require orthodontics or reconstruction.

How a Nonworking-Side Interference Harms the Teeth

There are many complex problems of the nonworking-side interference. Here we want to consider just the tooth.

The nonworking-side interference usually occurs on the last teeth in the arch. Because of the nonworking-side contact, the horizontal force pushes the lower tooth in a distobuccal direction. There is no proximal contact distal to the last lower tooth in the arch. This is a difficult area to keep clean (Fig. 40). Since the area is dirty and since there is no tooth distal to help take the force, the periodontium gives way. Examine patients for deep distobuccal pockets on the last lower molar. You may find

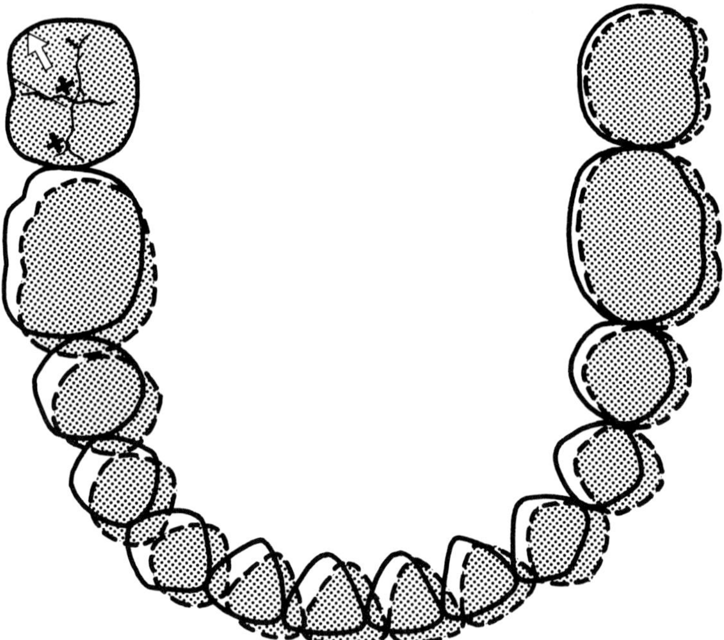

Fig. 40. Lower teeth in solid black outline indicate the MICP of teeth. Lower teeth in broken outline and shaded indicate lateral movement of lower teeth. X's indicate nonworking interference on right second molar. Arrow indicates direction of force of nonworking-side interference on right second molar. Note that since direction of force of nonworking-side contact is distobuccally, right second molar has lost its contact mesially with right first molar.

a number of them. Be sure to examine both sides of the dentition for nonworking-side interferences. Adjust both sides, if necessary, before placing a restoration. We suggest that at this point you start to examine patients for nonworking-side interferences. Eliminate all that you find. Practicing this procedure will give you valuable experience in:

1. Using articulating ribbon

2. Working with the patient and getting him to move the mandible the way you desire

3. Grinding away interferences and reexamining to be sure you did the job correctly

4. Gaining confidence

It makes no difference that you are not doing a complete occlusal adjustment. Eliminating the nonworking-side interferences is a good and safe way to get your fingers wet in occlusal adjustment.

A QUICK LOOK AT NONWORKING-SIDE INTERFERENCES

1. Where do nonworking-side interferences usually occur? *Between the molars on the nonworking side.*

2. Can nonworking-side interferences occur in the bicuspids also? *Yes, but not so frequently as in the molar area.*

3. Where do the markings from nonworking-side interferences occur? *On the distal inner inclines of the upper lingual cusps and on the mesial inner inclines of the lower buccal cusps, except in crossbite occlusions.*

4. Where should you usually grind to eliminate a nonworking-side interference? *On a distal inner incline of an upper lingual cusp.*

5. What about the crossbite occlusion? *For now try to master the more common situation. The same principles apply to the crossbite occlusion. All that is necessary is to think it through, applying the principles you have just learned.*

Elimination of the Working-Side Interference:
The Index Tooth and the Lateral Index

All lateral interferences must be ground away. First, however, a lateral interference must be identified. The key to the identification is the use of a lateral index.

A marginal ridge contacted by an opposing cusp tip during a lateral jaw movement is a naturally occurring lateral index. A cuspal incline that is contacted in a lateral movement but that has been reshaped so that the plane of contact is parallel to and continuous with the plane of that tooth's marginal ridge is an artificially prepared lateral index. Both of these are lateral indices because both are consistent with lateral freedom, as illustrated in Figure 29. (This assumes reasonably correct axial inclinations of the upper teeth.)

THE WORKING-SIDE INTERFERENCE, THE LATERAL INDEX, AND THE INDEX TOOTH.   To repeat, the key to the identification of the lateral interference lies in the marginal ridges of the upper cuspids and posterior teeth (assuming reasonably correct axial inclination).

A lateral bruxing jaw movement occurs when a person keeps his teeth in contact while moving his mandible laterally. Figures 29 and 31 show that, unless interfered with by opposing cusps, *the neuromuscular mechanism moves the lower teeth at an angle corresponding approximately to the marginal ridges of the opposing upper teeth.*

A lateral interference is any cuspal incline that contacts during a lateral jaw movement and causes its opposing tooth to move at an angle steeper than that of the adjacent marginal ridge. The mandible must open down and around this interference during lateral movement.

A lateral index, on the other hand, is a part of an upper tooth which, when contacted by lower cusps during a lateral movement, allows the neuromuscular mechanism to move the mandibular teeth sideward at an angle no greater than the marginal ridges of their opposing upper teeth. Thus, if an upper marginal ridge were contacted by a lower cusp tip during a lateral movement, it would form a naturally occurring lateral index.

However, in almost all natural occlusions, when the mandible moves sideward, the lower cusps will be contacting upper cuspal inclines and not upper marginal ridges. For an upper incline (which is a lateral interference) to be turned into a lateral index, it must be reshaped to allow the neuromuscular mechanism to move the mandible and lower teeth laterally at the same angle as that of the opposing upper marginal ridges.

An upper tooth that makes MICP contact and is capable of contact throughout the range of lateral motion can be ground and adjusted so that it has no lateral interferences. Such a tooth is referred to as an *index tooth*. The area of lateral contact is ground to an angle or plane corresponding to that of the marginal ridge. This prepared area on the *index tooth* can be used as a *lateral index* to determine lateral interferences on all the rest of the teeth on the working side.

Preparation of the index usually results in loss of contact of the index tooth during lateral motion. The reason is that the rest of the teeth on the working side, which have not been ground, are now contacting during lateral motion. With the use of articulating ribbon, these areas can be marked and ground. The marking and grinding process continues until only the index tooth marks throughout the range of lateral bruxing motion. The patient then has a free, unrestrained lateral movement without interference. During chewing there is no significant lateral contact between the teeth. While the index tooth is capable of contact during lateral movements, contact is unlikely unless the patient habitually bruxes. And bruxism is unlikely because the lateral index is not restraining. A lateral pathway has been provided for the patient.

SELECTION OF THE INDEX TOOTH.   To apply the lateral index an index tooth is needed. The index tooth guides in the elimination of all lateral interferences.

The index tooth must meet certain requirements. First, it must contact in the MICP and be capable of contact throughout lateral motion. Lateral interferences in the first instant of jaw motion are very damaging. It is during the initial part or instant of jaw motion that the muscles exert their greatest force. *People are most aware of interferences in the initial part of jaw movement.* Since these interferences make people brux, it is important that they be detected and eliminated.

The only way to see or record a lateral jaw movement in the mouth is to record it on the teeth. On articulators there are incisal guide tables that guide in waxing or setting teeth, and index teeth are just like these incisal guide tables. To get a complete recording from the MICP throughout lateral motion, it is necessary for the index tooth to contact in the MICP and be capable of contact throughout lateral motion.

Place the articulating ribbon between the teeth and have the patient close in the MICP and then rub his teeth together on the ribbon throughout lateral movement. Be sure the teeth are dry, and use dry ribbon whenever marking teeth.

The line or smudge made on the index tooth by the opposing cusp represents a record of lateral jaw movement on that tooth. It is the adjusting of this mark and then the adjusting of the other teeth to this mark that enable the dentist to create a lateral pathway.

The cuspid is the preferred tooth to use as an index tooth. It usually contacts in the MICP in an occlusion that requires adjusting. As will be discussed later, the last step is the elimination of anterior tooth contact in the MICP. For now, maintain MICP contact on the cuspid if it is present. (The reasons for using the cuspids as index teeth are discussed in detail on page 55.)

Another important requirement for the beginner at occlusal adjustments is that he select an index tooth that is firm. (A dentist experienced in occlusal adjustment can use a mobile tooth as an index tooth since if he adjusts the occlusion to perfection, the patient will no longer brux or contact the teeth in lateral movements.) If the cuspid is loose or does not contact in the MICP, then use the most anterior posterior firm tooth that makes contact in the MICP and that is capable of continuous contact during lateral motion.

To review:

1. The index tooth should contact in the MICP.

2. The index tooth should be capable of continuous contact during lateral jaw movement.

3. The index tooth should be firm.

4. The cuspid is preferred if it meets the other criteria.

Try to select an index tooth whose index is on the mesial half of the tooth. If the index is made on the distal half of an upper buccal cusp, it is on a holding or distal incline. Patients may remember indices on holding inclines and thus be more likely to brux. If the index is made on a mesial inner incline of an upper buccal cusp, the patient still has freedom to the border positions and will tend not to remember the index. If the index is forgotten, so is the habit of bruxing. However, in Angle Class II occlusion, often the index must be made on distal inclines. This requires more grinding so as to create the necessary freedom. Figure 41 elucidates the disadvantage of the Class II occlusion.

Why is an index tooth selected in this way? *Ideally, the result of an occlusal adjustment will be no tooth contact during lateral jaw movement.* Realistically, however, lateral tooth contacts do occur. With this in mind, the dentist seeks maximum safety for the index tooth and the patient's dentition and so selects and adjusts the index tooth carefully.

The cuspid is preferred because it is big and strong. It has the longest root, and if it gets hit once in a while, chances are it can take it. Also, the cuspid has only one root. Horizontal forces on furcated teeth crush the bone in the furcation. The bone in the depth of a furcation cannot adapt because it is confined in unyielding root structure. Bone around a single-rooted tooth does not have the same problem.

One other reason for selecting the cuspid is that it is farther from the temporomandibular joint. The farther the resistance from the joint in a second-class lever system, the less the mechanical advantage. In other words, the muscles can exert more power on the more posterior tooth and less power on the more anterior tooth. (There is still another safety factor that the cuspid possesses. It will be discussed later, when the anterior teeth come to our attention.)

Once the index tooth has been selected, it must be adjusted. For the sake of discussion, let us talk about upper cuspids as the index teeth. Other teeth would be adjusted the same way, but the cuspid is the one most often used.

Lateral motion is adjusted as described below. Remember that

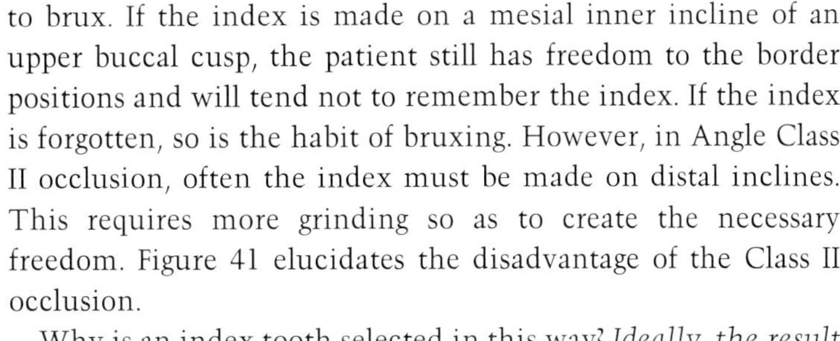

FIG. 41. *A,* Class I occlusion. Lower cusps enter and leave mesial fossae of upper teeth. Upper buccal cusps are not in path of lateral movement. *B,* Class II occlusion. Lower buccal cusps enter and leave distal fossae of upper teeth. Upper buccal cusps interfere with path of lateral movement of lower cusps. Note that cuspid and bicuspid area interferes with lateral movement more than molars do. This happens because there is a greater protrusive component to lateral movement in cuspid and bicuspid area of dental arch. The asterisk-like mark indicates lateral interference.

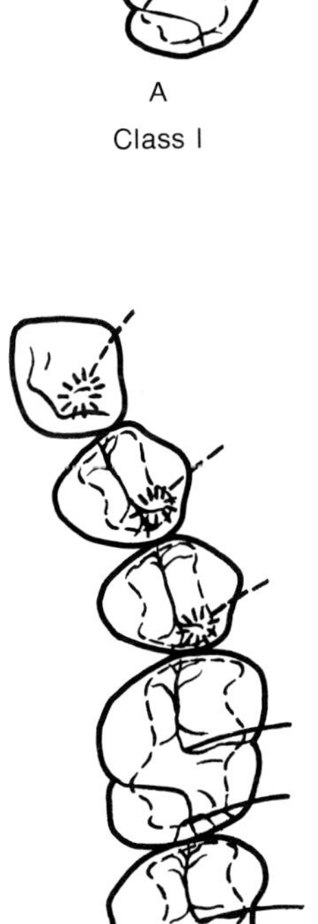

A

Class I

B

Class II

all nonworking-side interferences have already been checked and eliminated.

EXAMINATION.   Mark the teeth. Dry the teeth on the working side and place articulating ribbon between them. Have the patient close on the ribbon and move his jaw from side to side a couple of times. Make sure he rubs his teeth against one another during this movement. The interferences on the working side occur between the outer inclines of the supporting cusps and the inner inclines of the nonsupporting cusps (Fig. 42).

Tell the patient to open and remain open while you examine the marks. If the patient closes and swallows, the marks will be washed away and the marking procedure must be repeated.

Examine the mark on the index tooth. If the index tooth only has a mark indicating contact in the MICP, some other tooth is contacting during the lateral movement and causing the index tooth to separate. The example case, delineated in Figures 43 and 44, shows this very situation, which is not a common one.

IDENTIFYING OCCLUSAL MARKINGS.   Figure 43 shows schematically how the example case marks. Note that the occlusal relationship illustrated is cusp-to-fossa. Each cusp tip and opposing

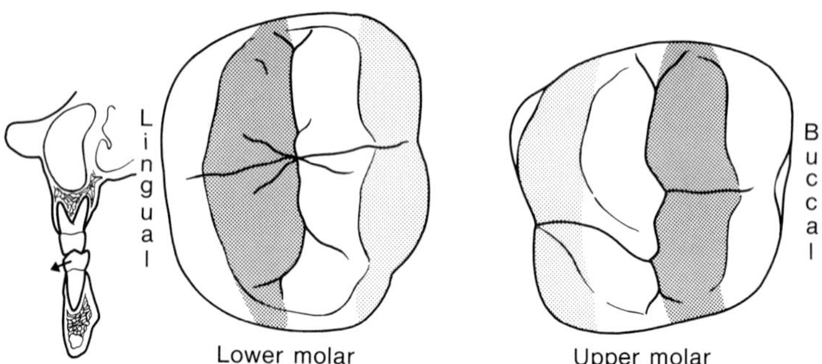

FIG. 42. Darkly shaded inclines are inner inclines of nonsupporting cusps (upper buccal and lower lingual). Lightly shaded areas are outer inclines of supporting cusps (lower buccal and upper lingual). Interferences on working side occur between outer inclines of supporting cusps and inner inclines of nonsupporting cusps. In adjustment of working side, most grinding will be done on inner inclines of nonsupporting cusps. Grinding inner inclines of nonsupporting cusps increases range of motion for supporting cusps. However, if supporting cusps are worn and flat, their outer inclines should also be ground. Do *not* grind away point area that will become cusp tip and contact opposing tooth in MICP.

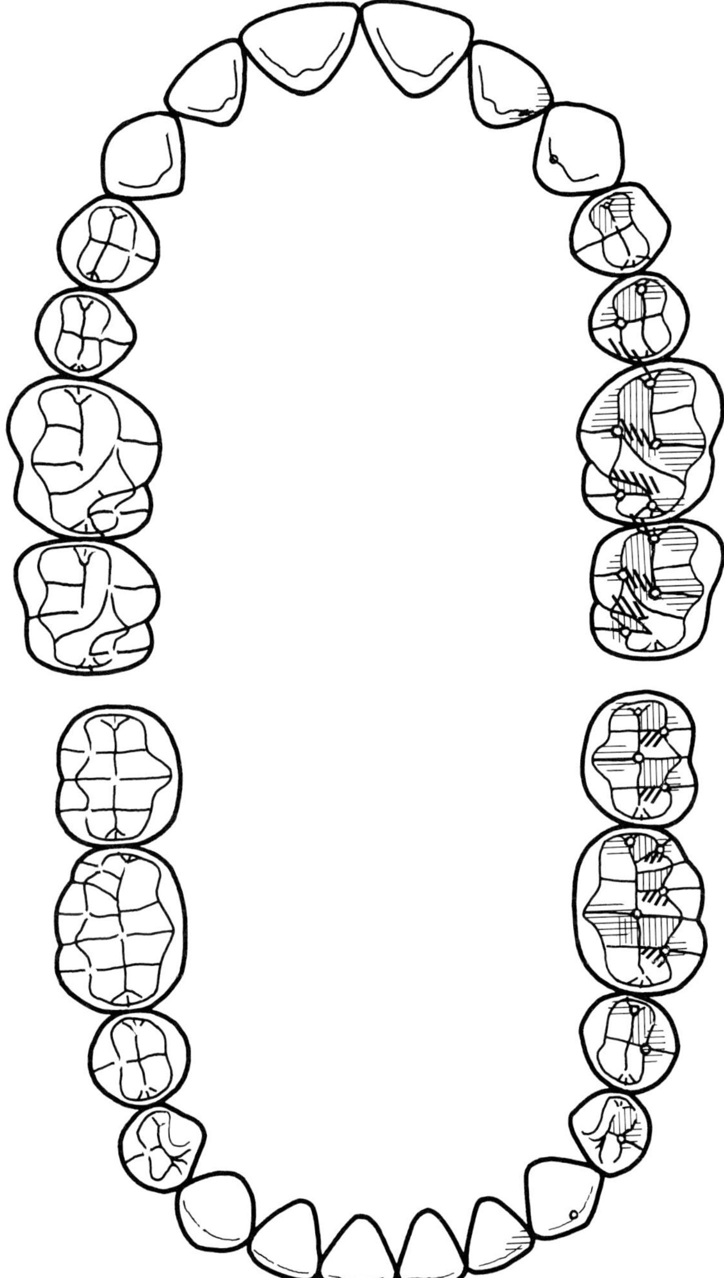

FIG. 43. Example case marked. Vertical lines represent centric relation interferences; horizontal lines, lateral interferences; and oblique lines, non-working-side interferences. From this assortment of marks you must pick out the marks you need—the MICP contacts, the white circles on the supporting cusp tips and in their opposing fossae.

fossa has marked. In reality this seldom occurs, except in a severely worn dentition. In addition to marking lateral interferences, you cannot help but mark centric interferences and perhaps you will also mark the nonworking-side interferences. For now, do not dwell on figuring out the centric adjustment of the occlusion. (Pages 107–112 cover centric adjustment in detail.) At this time, we want only to explain the marks and what to do with them.

If the supporting cusps are severely worn and if there are smudges from lateral contact on their mesial and distal slopes, reshape these slopes (Fig. 44). The cusp tip may also be worn and widened mesiodistally. If it is, the buccal and lingual inclines of the cusp should also be reshaped and in such a way that the part of the flattened cusp that will become the cusp tip is as close as possible to the opposing fossa.

Do not grind the MICP markings at the bases of the fossa and marginal-ridge areas or on the tips of supporting cusps. In many instances, the supporting cusps may be suspended in their opposing fossae, requiring special consideration in adjustment (see Fig. 54).

TECHNIQUE (PRELIMINARY). *Beginning the Lateral Grind.*

Study the marks on the teeth and pick out the contact spots that represent MICP contacts. Make a mental picture of them. These are the marks you must *not* grind. (They are the small white circles in Figure 43.) They are the tips of the supporting cusps and the fossa and marginal-ridge areas they contact.

I. Grind all marks on the inner inclines of the upper and lower supporting cusps (the lower buccal and upper lingual cusps). These marks are centric and nonworking-side interferences. (In Figure 43, the centric interferences are shown as vertical lines and the nonworking-side interferences as oblique lines.) Even though you are not doing a centric adjustment at this time, you can safely grind these inclines during the lateral adjustment. *Do not* grind the contact dot nor the holding boundary just mesial to it on an upper tooth or just distal to it on a lower tooth.

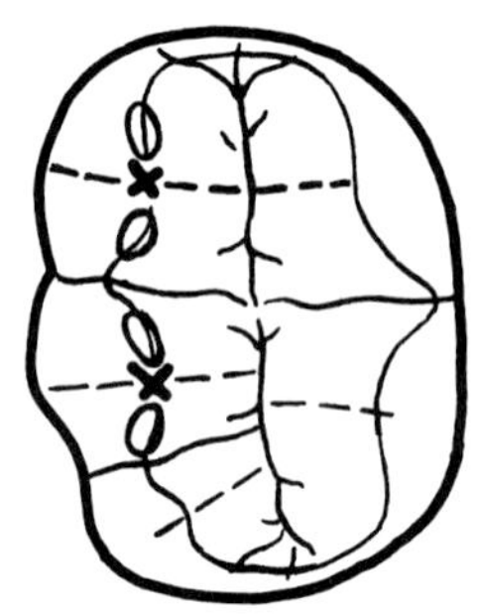

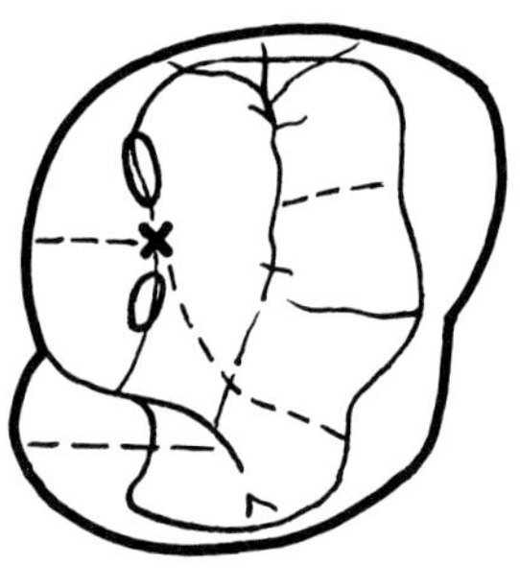

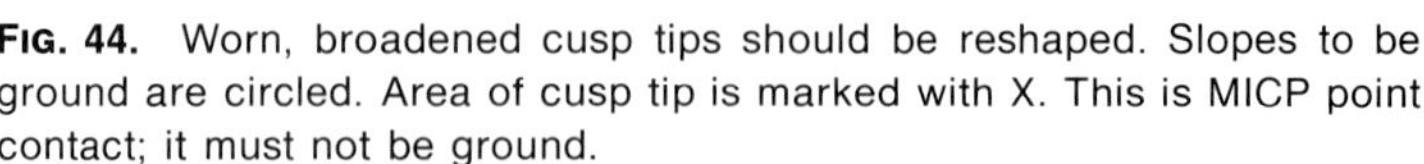

FIG. 44. Worn, broadened cusp tips should be reshaped. Slopes to be ground are circled. Area of cusp tip is marked with X. This is MICP point contact; it must not be ground.

II. Grind all marks on the inner inclines of the upper and lower nonsupporting cusps (the upper buccal and lower lingual cusps). These are lateral interferences. (In Figure 43 they are shown as horizontal lines.)

   Note again that the cuspids contact in the MICP but do not contact during lateral movement. By grinding the teeth as just mentioned, you will get the cuspids to contact during lateral movement.

III. If the anterior teeth strike and mark during lateral movement, grind the lingual surface of the upper anterior tooth. Do not grind the very tip of the mark nearest the palate, since this part of the mark represents MICP contact. It will be removed eventually but not at this point. If there is a deep overbite and the incisors continue to interfere during lateral movements, the deep overbite will have to be adjusted (pp. 97–99).

IV. After completing this amount of grinding (we use a #110 diamond wheel or one slightly larger—never a smaller one), mark the teeth again, as before. Since you have ground the working side, look to the other side of the mouth—there may now be some nonworking-side interferences. So, before re-marking the teeth on the working side, mark the nonworking side and look for nonworking-side interferences. This is a common situation; Figure 45 shows nonworking-side interferences (*oblique lines*) along with the re-marking of the working side.

V. Grind away the marks of the nonworking-side interferences. Do not grind away the MICP contact spots. If necessary, refer to the section on the adjustment of the nonworking side (pp. 43–46).

VI. Grind on the working side as before and as just described. Repeat the checking and adjusting of the nonworking-side interferences as well, and keep marking and adjusting the working side until the index tooth is the only tooth contacted during lateral movement.

   The results of the grinding in the example case are shown in Figure 46. Since the index tooth (in this case, the upper cuspid) did not contact during lateral movement initially, we could not adjust it. But now it is the only

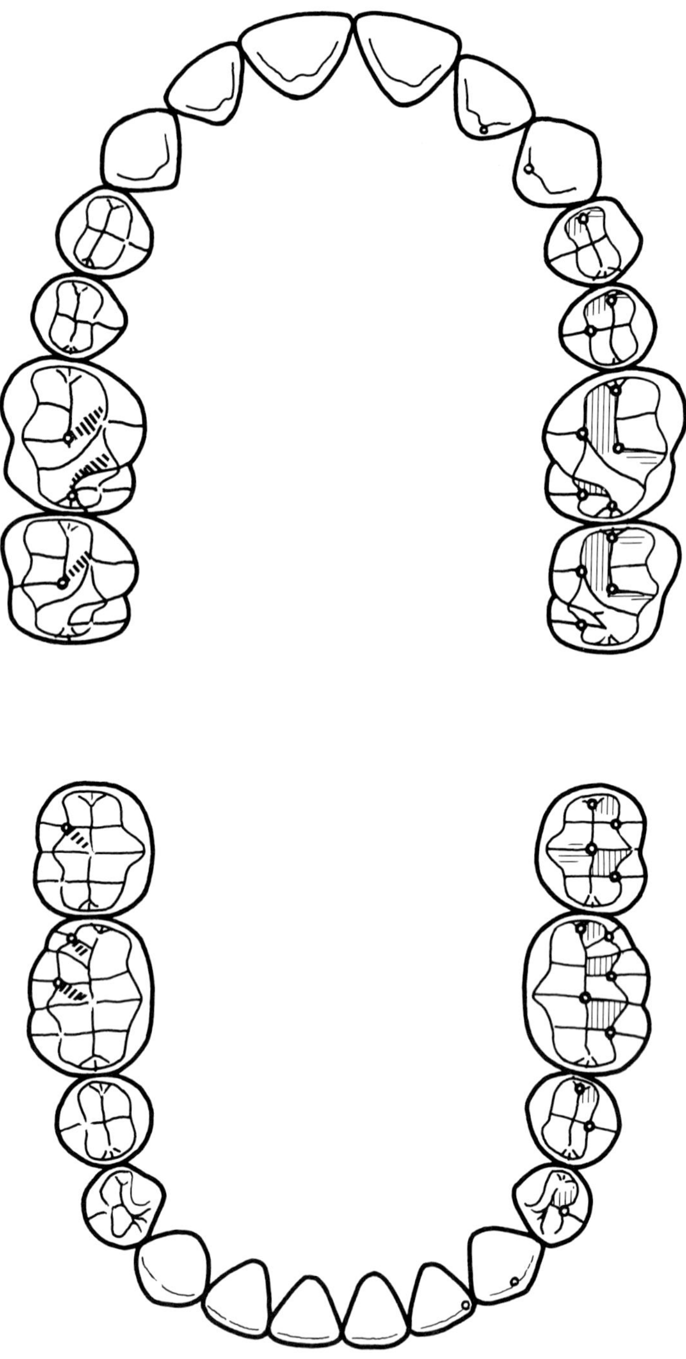

FIG. 45. Re-marking after initial lateral grinding. There are now interferences on nonworking side (*oblique lines on opposite side of arch*), and interferences still remain on working side.

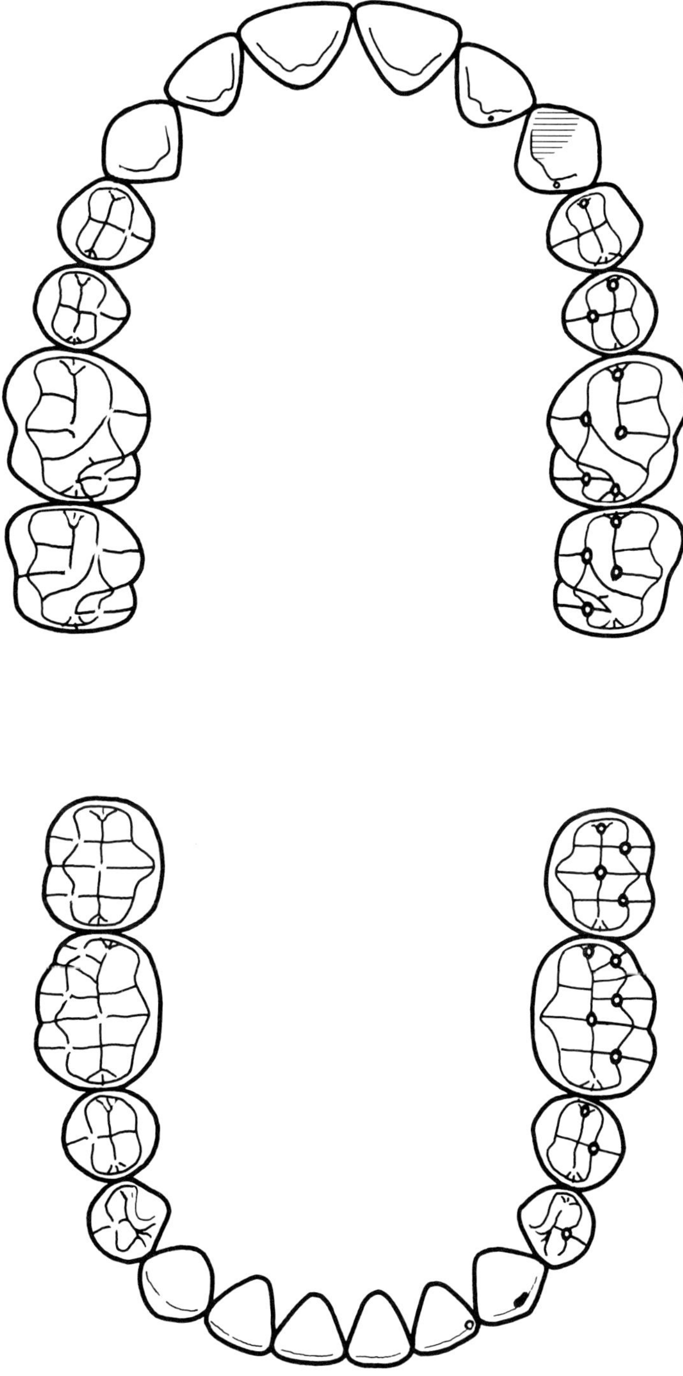

FIG. 46. All lateral interferences have been removed. Contact during lateral movement can now occur only on cuspid (index tooth).

tooth that contacts during lateral movement, and it can be adjusted. If the index tooth had contacted during the original lateral movement, as is usually the case, we would have adjusted it as the first step in the lateral adjustment.

ADJUSTING THE INDEX TOOTH.   Most of the marking or smudge on the index tooth represents a record of the lateral movement of the lower cuspid. The very tip of the mark or smudge closest to the palate represents the MICP contact.

You may also see a mark on the upper cuspid made by the lower first bicuspid or lower lateral incisor. The lower first bicuspid may make a mark on the distal inner slope of the upper cuspid, and the lower lateral incisor may make a mark on the mesial inner slope of the upper cuspid.

To have unrestrained lateral movement, the mark of lateral contact on the index tooth must be at the optimal angle, the smallest angle possible with the horizontal plane. In reviewing what was said in Figures 29 and 31 about the lateral index and lateral movement, it becomes apparent that a reasonable angle to create for lateral movement on the index tooth is the angle of the tooth's marginal ridge. Naturally this assumes that the tooth has a reasonably correct axial inclination.

If the line or smudge representing lateral movement is not on the same plane as that of the marginal ridge (Fig. 47A), grind the area and blend it into the plane of the marginal ridge. When the lower tooth moves mesiodistally across the index tooth, as it sometimes does, the index tooth may be hollow ground or concave when finished.

Grind the entire area of the line or smudge, but *do not grind the very tip of the mark nearest the palate*. The amount of the mark retained should be as small as possible (Fig. 47B). This is the MICP part of the mark and it must be retained for now. This part of the mark is the last thing to be adjusted. (It will be discussed later, when adjustment of the anterior teeth is considered.)

Grind not only the mark from lateral movement but also the surrounding areas mesially and distally so that the grinding blends with the remainder of the cusp. Grind until the surface of the cuspid you are working on is on the same plane as that of the marginal-ridge area of the tooth. Remember that the mark or recording of lateral motion on the index tooth (upper cuspid) may not be directionally parallel with the marginal ridge (and

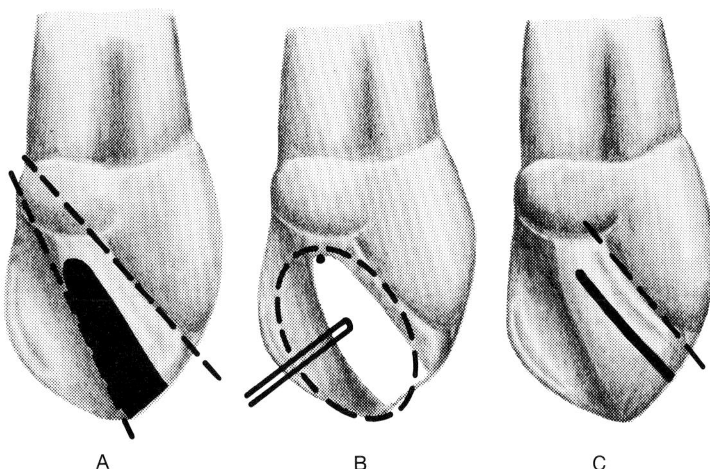

FIG. 47. *A,* Lateral contact mark on index tooth is at angle steeper than that of marginal ridge. *B,* Marked incline is ground until it is on plane parallel to that of marginal ridge. Note that tiny MICP contact is *not* ground. *C,* Lateral contact mark is now on incline that is parallel to marginal ridge.

most often it is not) but that the area marked should be adjusted by grinding until it is on a plane parallel with that of the marginal ridge (Fig. 47C). Make sure that the surface you have adjusted is flat or concave and that it has no bumps in it. The lower cuspid cusp tip must ride on a flat or concave *smooth* surface from the beginning of lateral movement throughout the range of lateral movement.

Although the marginal ridge of an upper tooth is used to give a reasonable idea about the inclination of the lateral index, we do not mean to imply that the adjustment of the lateral index is a mechanical procedure. It is not.

After the adjustment has been completed, check for fremitus while the patient makes lateral bruxing movements. If fremitus is present, refine the index by making sure it is polished and smooth from the very minute point of MICP contact throughout the lateral movement. Sometimes this results in the index's having a concave course during the lateral bruxing movement. The important thing is that there be *no fremitus.*

The direction of the mark on the surface of the index tooth that represents the lateral movement of the lower cusp tip will not necessarily be parallel to the direction of the marginal ridge of the index tooth. Usually it is not parallel (Fig. 48).

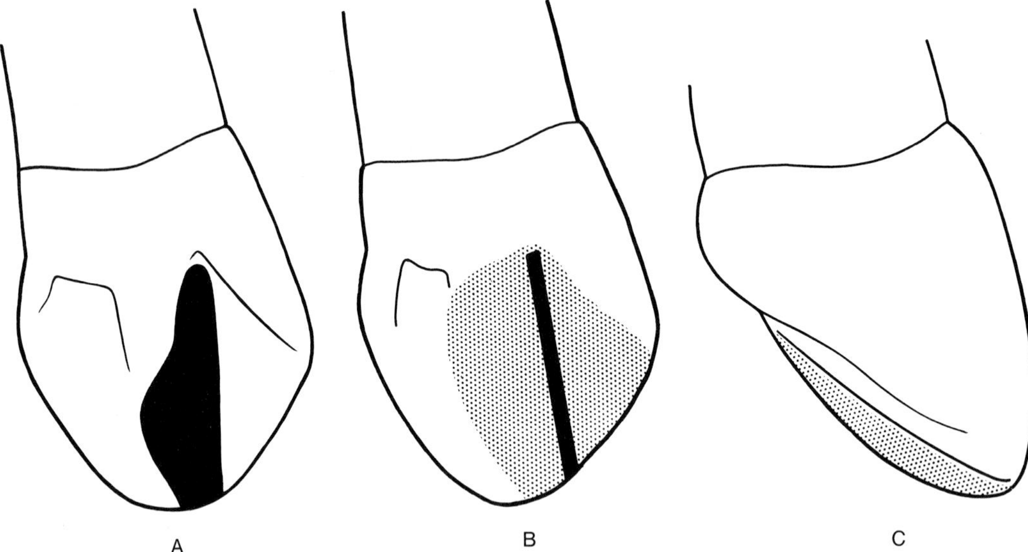

FIG. 48. *A,* Mark made on upper cuspid (index tooth) by lower cuspid during lateral movement is mesiodistally in direction different from marginal ridge. *B,* Wide mark of lateral movement reduced to narrow line. *C,* Mesial view. Even though mark of lateral contact is not parallel to marginal ridge mesiodistally, it is on plane parallel to that of marginal ridge.

The adjustment of the index tooth makes the plane of the index surface the same as or parallel to the plane of the marginal ridge. When all lateral interferences have been ground away, the index tooth will be the only tooth to mark during a lateral bruxing movement.

A Common Mistake

When grinding a lateral interference, be sure to grind *all the way to the MICP mark.* Instead of just a hint or minute speck of MICP contact, often a millimeter or more is left during the adjustment (Fig. 49). This is a serious error. Leaving an interference on a posterior tooth during the first millimeter of lateral movement could cause the patient to brux. The discussion of the first requirement for an index tooth (p. 53) stressed how important it is to eliminate interferences during the initial part of a lateral movement.

If you are changing the angle of lateral movement on the cuspid from 60 degrees to 50 degrees with respect to the horizon, then it must be changed from the very beginning of the lateral

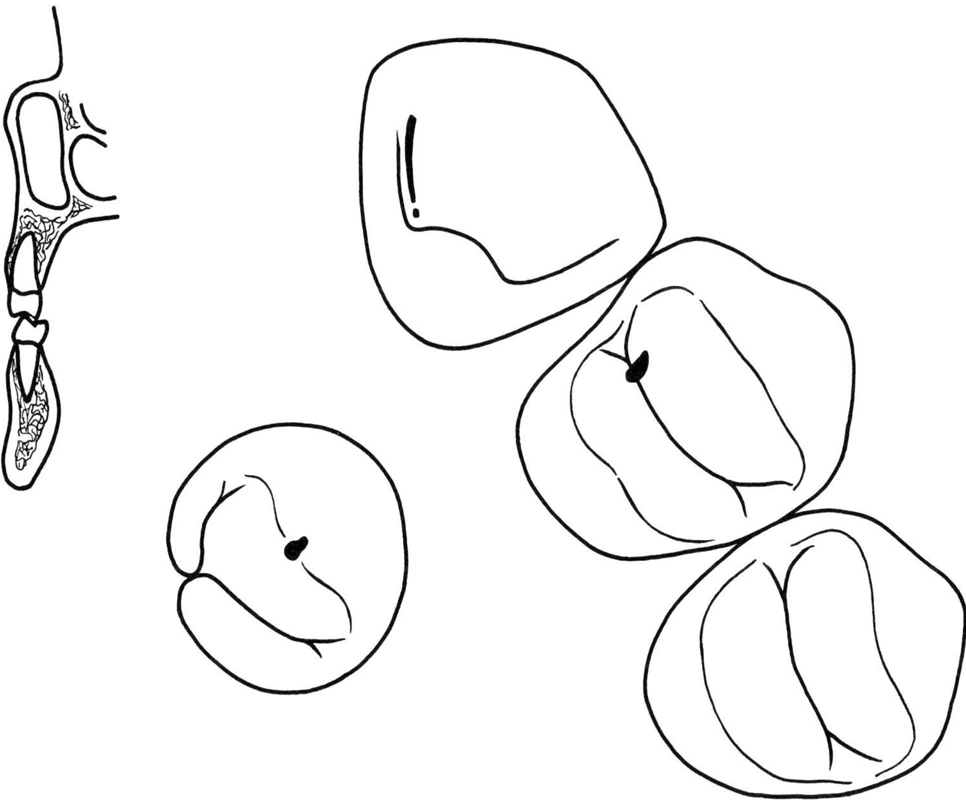

FIG. 49. A common mistake. First millimeter of lateral contact is still on posterior tooth because interfering incline on bicuspid was not ground all the way to MICP contact point. For first millimeter, bicuspid is in contact and cuspid (index tooth) is not.

movement. It is incorrect to have the initial part or millimeter of the movement on the index tooth at 60 degrees and then go to 50 degrees (Figs. 47C, 50). The part of the movement at 60 degrees is still an interference. A lateral pathway has not been established until the entire lateral movement, including the initial and most important part of that movement, is at a reasonable angle.

Once the index tooth has been adjusted, the difficult part of the lateral adjustment is over. Realize that immediately after adjusting the index tooth it may no longer contact in lateral motion. Perhaps the reason is that the other teeth are contacting during lateral movement, causing the index tooth to separate. If that is the case, further adjustment is required.

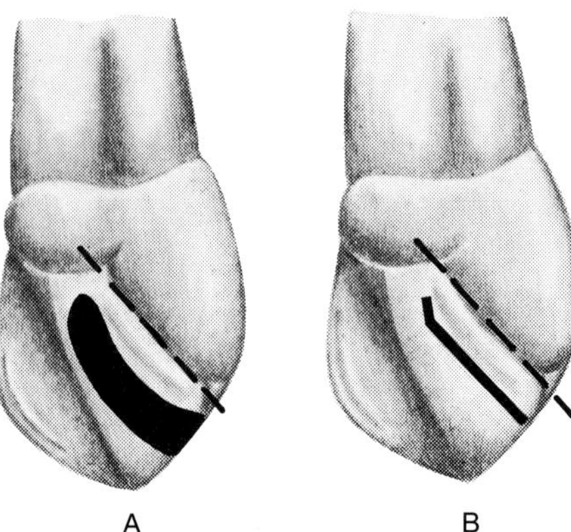

A   B

FIG. 50. _A,_ Large smudge of lateral contact on cuspid. **_B,_** Incorrect adjustment of lateral index. First millimeter of contact is still on plane steeper than that of marginal ridge. Properly completed lateral index should look like that in Fig. 47C.

TECHNIQUE. _Completing the Lateral Grind._

Figure 46 shows the sample case with only the cuspid making lateral contact. Figure 51 shows the sample case re-marked after the index tooth has been adjusted. Since the index tooth has been ground, it no longer contacts during lateral movement. The inner inclines of other upper buccal cusps and lower lingual cusps now contact during lateral jaw movement. These are interferences that prevent the lower tooth from contacting the index of the index tooth.

Grind all the marks of lateral contact or interferences as described before. In other words, grind away the marks on the inner inclines of the nonsupporting cusps right to the pinpoint MICP contact. The pinpoint MICP contact is not removed.

If for any reason the inner inclines of the nonsupporting cusps cannot be ground, the facial slopes of the supporting cusps can be ground. However, the very tip of the supporting cusp, which is the MICP contact, is _not_ ground.

In the example case, after the above adjustment, the re-marking might look like that in Figure 52. Note that the index tooth needs further refinement. The broad smudge should be refined to a line by grinding the area farthest from the nearest marginal ridge. In this case, the nearest marginal ridge is the mesial marginal ridge of the upper cuspid. Therefore, grind the distal portion of the mark. The result of this refinement is seen in Figure 53.

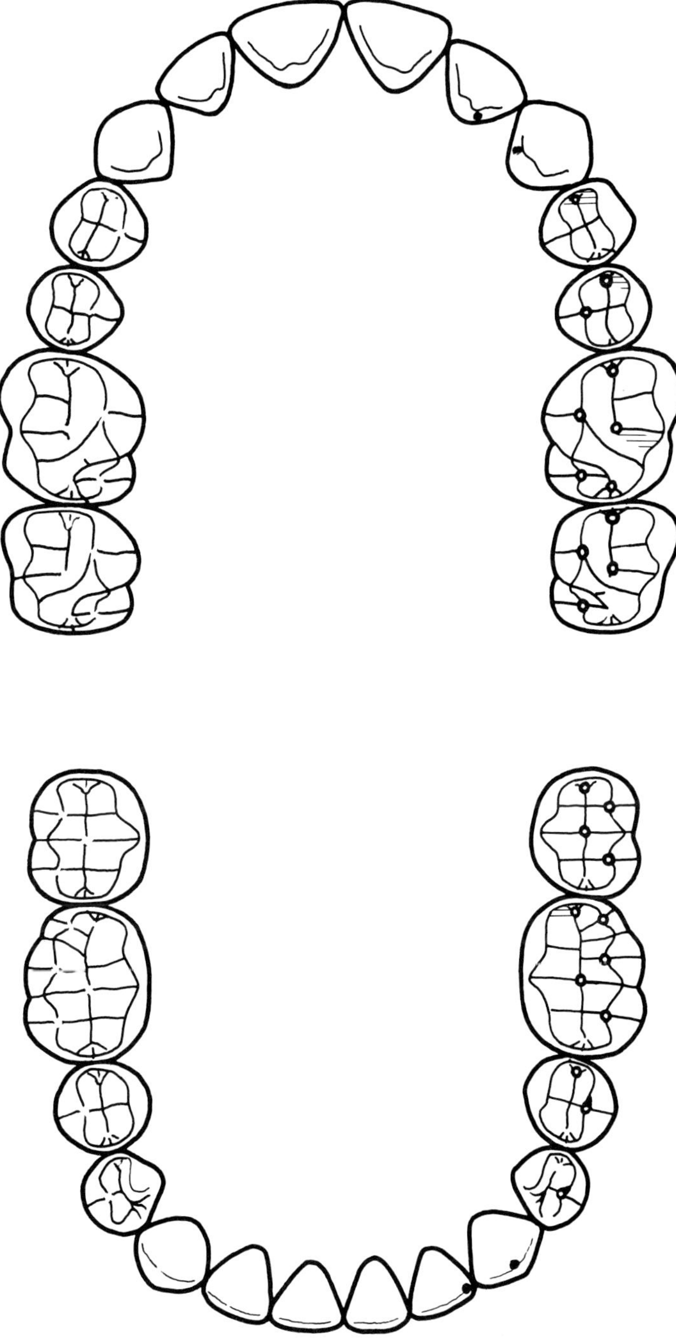

FIG. 51. Re-marking after grinding lateral index into index tooth. Index tooth (cuspid) no longer marks. There are lateral interferences (*horizontal lines*) on posterior teeth.

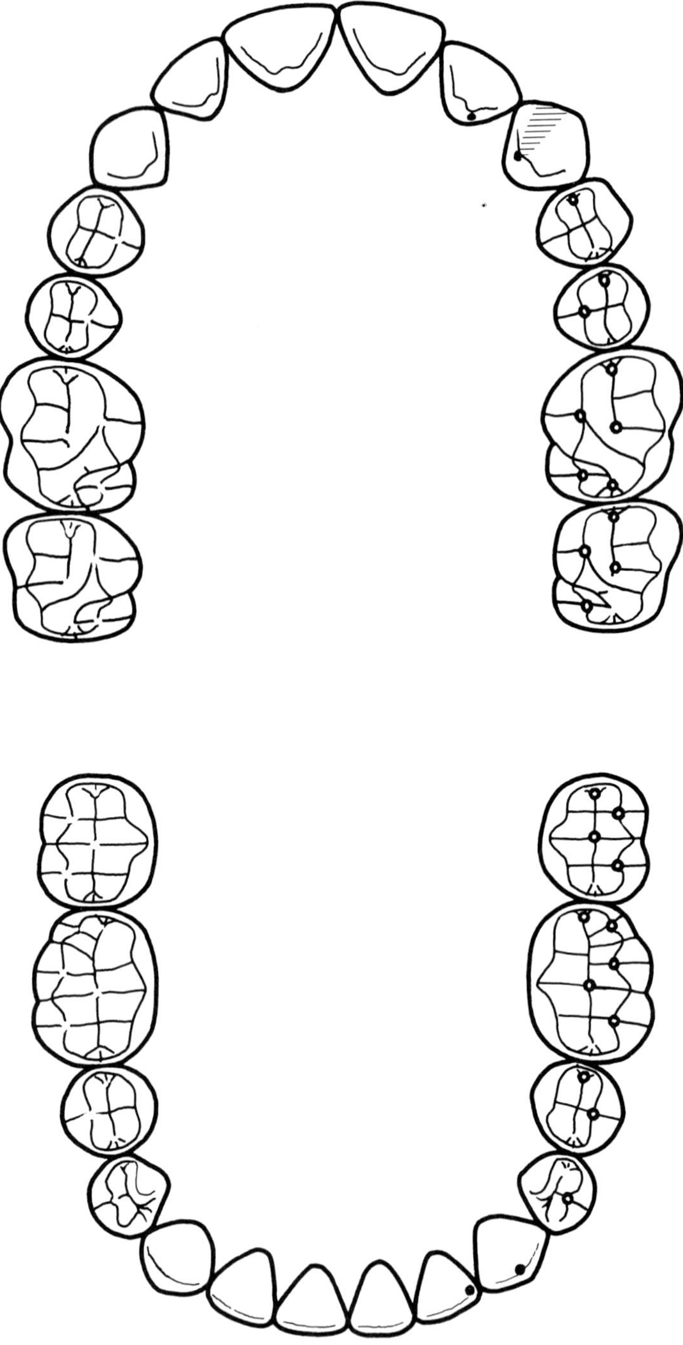

FIG. 52. Lateral interferences have been removed from posterior teeth. Only lateral index on index tooth now marks during lateral jaw movement. However, the mark is too broad.

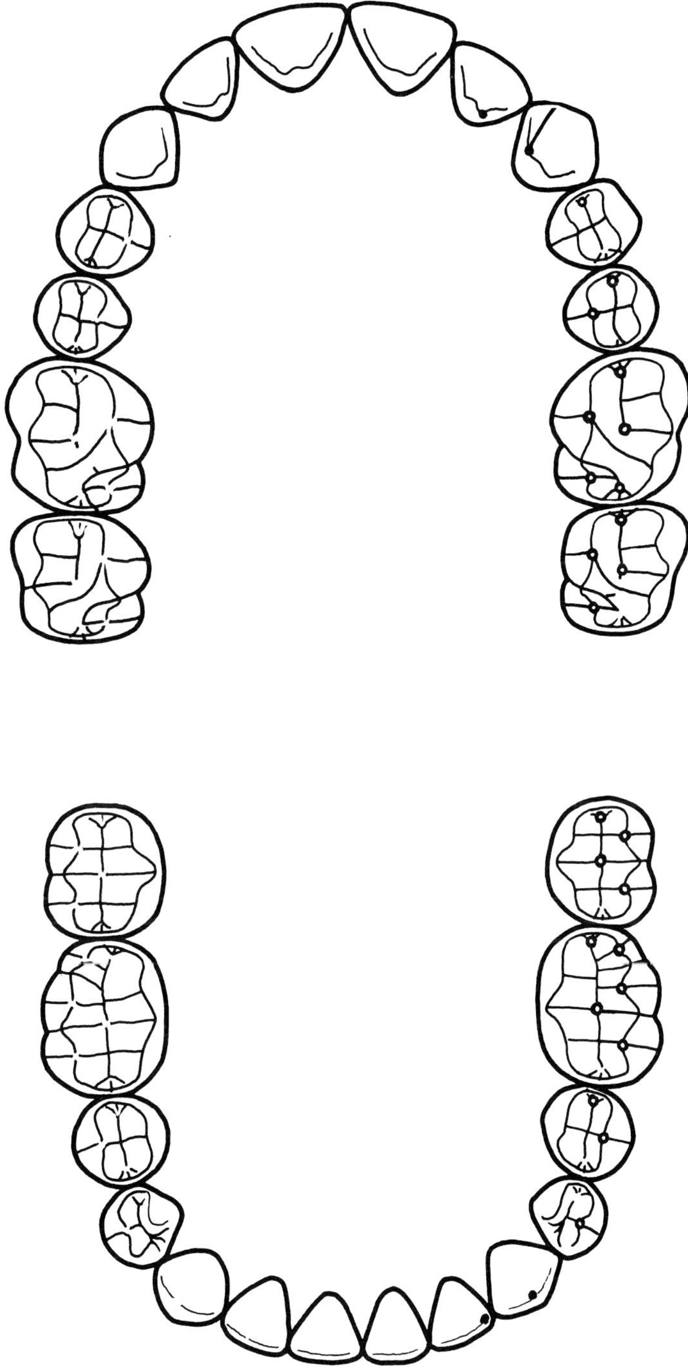

FIG. 53. Mark on index tooth is refined. However, MICP contacts are too large and need refining.

Figure 53 shows the completed lateral adjustment with one glaring error remaining, however. The error is that the MICP contacts are too large. They must be refined to pinpoint size. Keep the deepest pinpoint part of the mark, and polish the rest away.

The mark on the index tooth may not appear as a straight line. It may start out as a line but then develop into a smudge or wavy line. The reason is that when lateral movement is made, the lower cusp tip moves away from the flat or concave smooth plane established on the index tooth. Instead of the very tip of the lower cusp remaining in contact, the mesial or distal inclines begin to contact. When this happens, it is most often the distal incline of the lower cusp that separates the lower cusp tip from the previously established surface on the index tooth.

To remedy this, grind the smudge on the incline of the lower cusp. (Do not grind the tip of the lower cusp.) You can also grind the upper smudge, but, since the index tooth has already been adjusted and polished, it is often easier to make this adjustment on the lower tooth.

If the incisors are the only teeth contacting during lateral movements, adjust them as directed on pp. 95–100. After or during the lateral adjustment, check to make sure that you clear a lateral pathway to the border positions. This requires that you guide the patient's mandible distally while the patient makes lateral bruxing movements on the articulating paper or ribbon.

It is probably a good idea to do the lateral adjustment by first letting the patient make the lateral bruxing movements without guidance. Then, guide the patient's chin distally and toward the working side while he makes lateral bruxing movements with the ribbon between the teeth. There may now be marks of lateral interference in the *border movement* of the jaw. They should be eliminated to complete the lateral adjustment.

A lateral pathway has now been established for lateral movement to one side of the dentition. Next, repeat the entire procedure on the opposite side of the dentition.

There is no reason why you cannot practice lateral adjustment without doing or completing a centric adjustment. In fact, we suggest that occlusal adjustment be learned in stages. First, master the technique of placing restorations with cusp seats (pp. 16–25). Then master the technique for elimination of non-working-side interferences. After that, you are ready to start doing lateral adjustment. Learn occlusion in stages, and master each stage before proceeding to the next. Do not try to learn occlusal adjustment overnight—it cannot be done.

Management of the Multiple MICP Contact

In most of the illustrations in this book the MICP contacts are shown as single marks on the very tips of the supporting cusps and in the depths of the fossae. However, if there has been minimal wear of the teeth, the tips of the supporting cusps and the depths of the fossae will not touch and therefore not mark with articulating ribbon. The supporting cusp tips are suspended in the fossae and contact is made around the very tips of the cusps and pits of the fossae. So there may be two, three, or four marks of occlusal contact around the cusp tips and pits of the fossae (Fig. 54).

If these multiple marks of occlusal contact are smudges rather than pinpoint marks of contact, they should be adjusted. Occlusal contacts in the MICP should be pinpoint whether there is one contact between a cusp tip and fossa, multiple contacts between a cusp and fossa, or two contacts between a cusp and marginal ridges.

To do this adjustment, the pinpoint spots of the smudges nearest the pits of the fossae are retained. The remainder of the smudges around the pits of the fossae are ground out of contact. The smudges on the supporting cusp tips are not ground. The adjustment of these multiple smudges of occlusal contact is done only in the fossa areas. By adjusting in the fossa areas, you increase the freedom of movement of the supporting cusps.

Cusp-Seat Freedom and Lateral Motion

No matter what movement the mandible makes, the freedom area of the cusp seat insures that the opposing cusp tip will not run into any restraining cuspal inclines.

The cusp seat with its freedom area prevents any interference during a Bennett movement. The Bennett movement is a side shift of the working-side condyle at the beginning of a lateral movement. It affects primarily the first millimeter or so of lateral movement.

People have considerable muscle power in this first millimeter of lateral movement, and thus it is most important that no

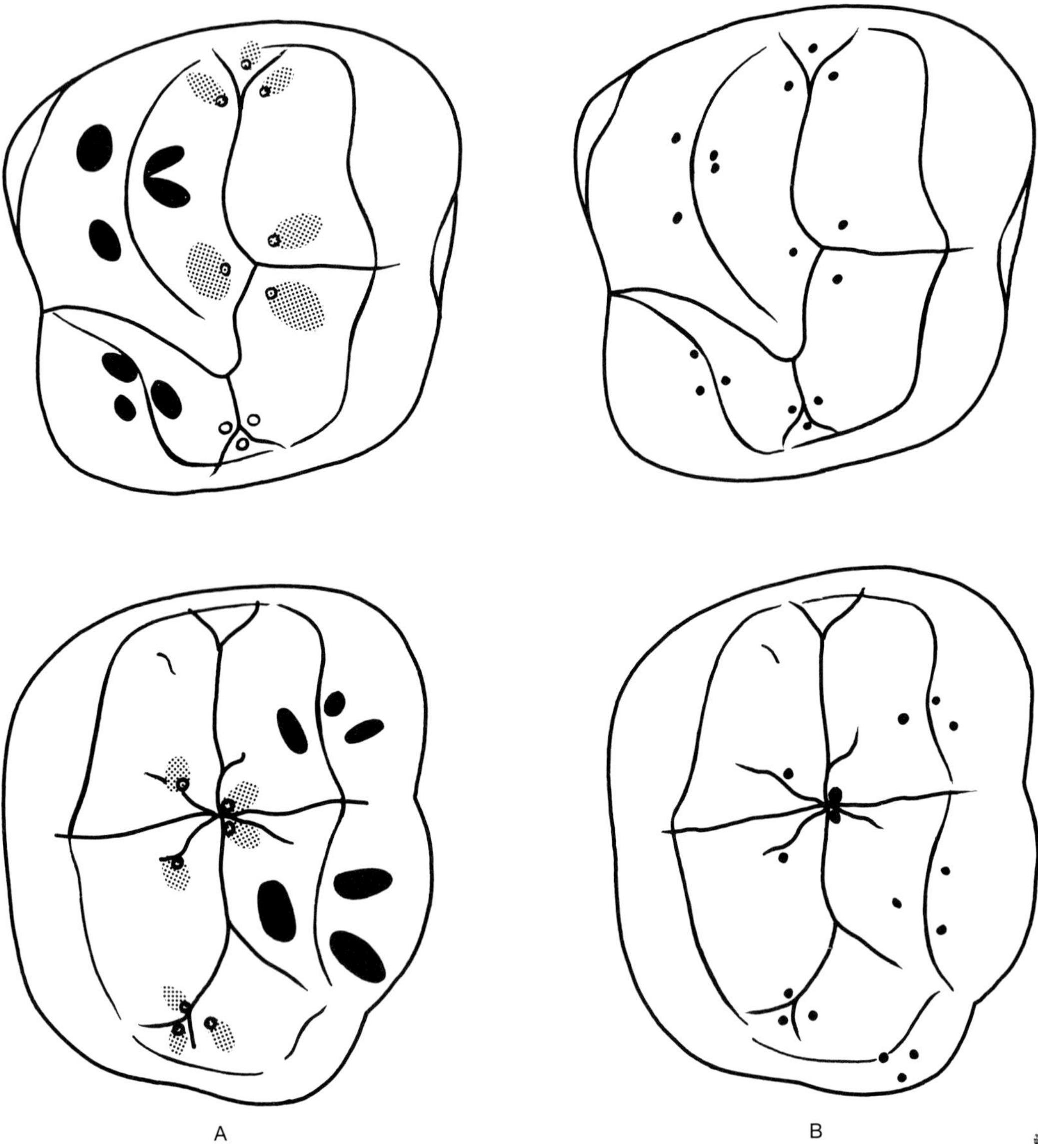

FIG. 54. **A,** Multiple smudges of MICP contact. Pinpoint contacts to be retained in fossae are circled. Dotted area is ground away. **B,** Result of adjustment: only pinpoint multiple contacts remain.

restraining cuspal incline should be contacted there. Restraint of Bennett movement in the molar area, which interferes with normal mandibular movement, can initiate bruxing, places great force on the teeth, and is particularly damaging. The freedom area of the cusp seat provides a Bennett miss-path, insuring that no posterior inclines are contacted during lateral jaw movement.

Establishment of the Lateral Index On an Upper Bicuspid

When an upper posterior tooth is being used as an index tooth, the only area that should mark during a lateral movement is a line (lateral index) that is on a plane parallel to the plane of the marginal ridge of that same posterior tooth.

This lateral index often takes a course up the cuspal incline in a direction quite different mesiodistally from the marginal ridge. The important thing is that, although the direction differs mesiodistally, it is on a plane parallel to that of the marginal ridge (Fig. 55). Also, the lateral index is a thin line rather than a broad smudge (Fig. 56C).

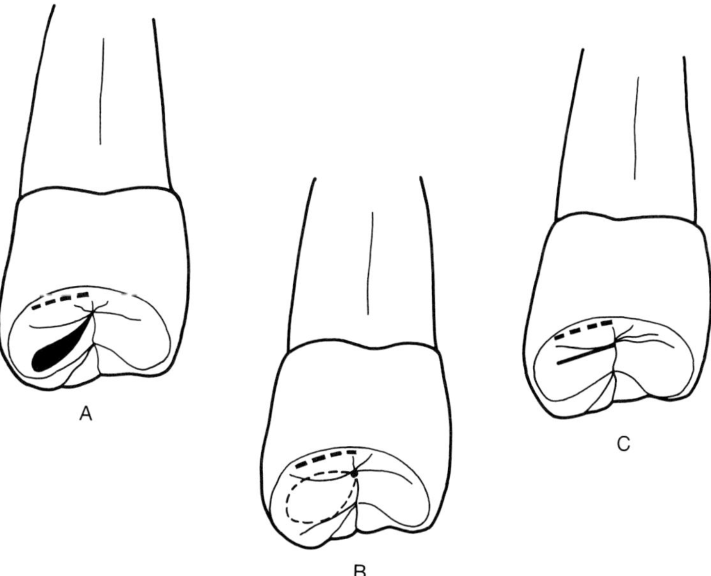

FIG. 55. Making lateral index on bicuspid. **A,** Mark of lateral contact is entirely on upper bicuspid cuspal incline. It is at much steeper angle than marginal-ridge area, which is represented by line of dashes. **B,** Entire mark is relieved, *except for MICP dot.* **C,** Upper incline is reshaped so that mark lower cusp tip now makes is thin line on a plane parallel to marginal-ridge area of tooth.

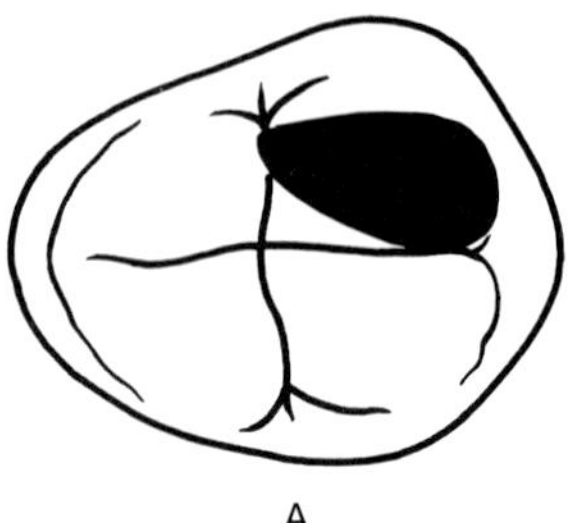
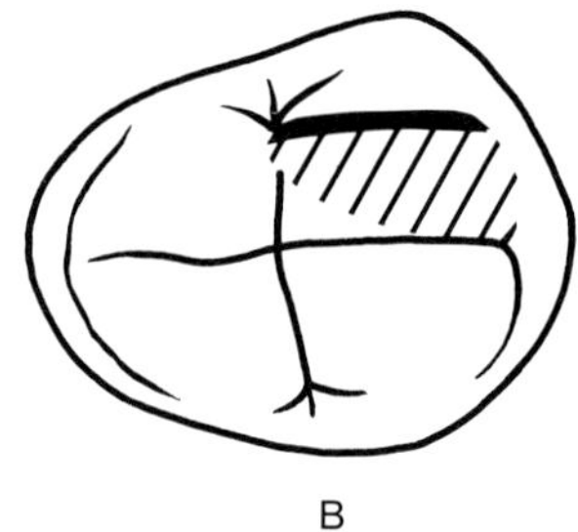
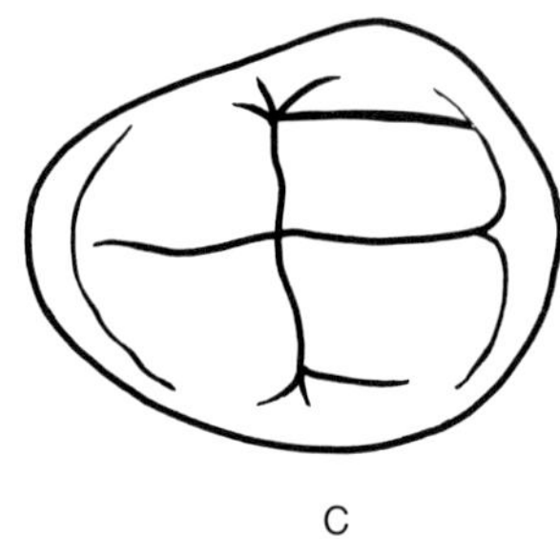

A   B   C

FIG. 56. Lateral index on bicuspid. *A,* Large smudge of lateral contact on inclines and on marginal-ridge area. *B,* Entire mark is relieved, except for MICP contact and thin line on marginal ridge. *C,* Lateral index is now thin line on marginal ridge.

RESTORATIONS CAN RESTRAIN AND CAN CAUSE TRAUMATOGENIC OCCLUSION

Restorations can cause immediate or delayed restraint. Immediate restraint can develop when a cement or a gutta percha temporary filling is being placed. It can also occur with permanent restorative materials.

Immediate restraint produces a sudden change in patient awareness and reaction. The immediate reaction is clenching or bruxing. An example of immediate restraint is a high filling that the patient notices the instant he occludes. Another is a cement or a gutta percha temporary filling that locks into a supporting cusp, causing lateral restraint even though it may not be high in the MICP. In either case the patient immediately bruxes his teeth (Fig. 57).

Delayed restraint is much more subtle and insidious in the way it brings about bruxing and traumatogenic occlusion. Since the restraint develops slowly, the patient is unaware of the changes taking place. Unless the dentist is aware of the importance of restraint, neither he nor the patient will suspect that a restoration placed months or years before can cause habitual bruxing and traumatogenic occlusion.

Delayed restraint occurs when restorations are overcarved and do not contact the opposing teeth. This condition produces instability of the teeth, and they shift or erupt into restraining contacts. The shifting or erupting may take months or years, but finally the delayed restraint develops and, along with it, bruxing and clenching (Fig. 58). Permanent restorations placed without an occlusal plan can lead to the collapse of the entire dentition.

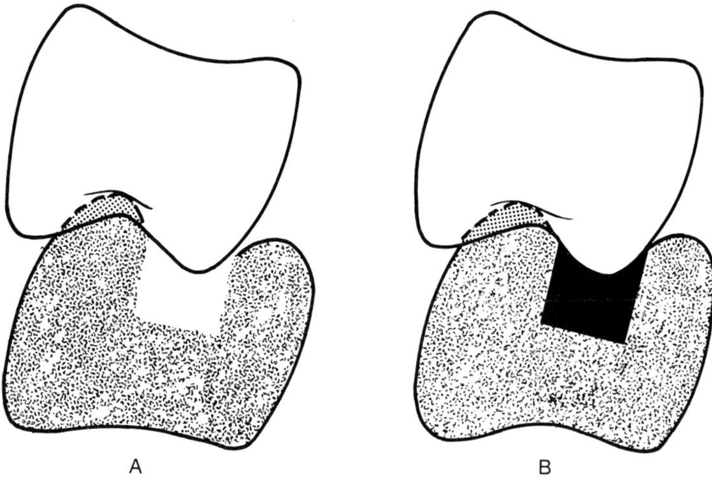

FIG. 57. Temporary restoration and restraint. **A,** Relationship before temporary restoration is placed. **B,** Cross-section through temporary restoration. (Temporary restoration shown in black.) Note that upper lingual cusp is "locked in"; no lateral movement is possible, and freedom is lost. Bruxing and general awareness of restoration can be expected.

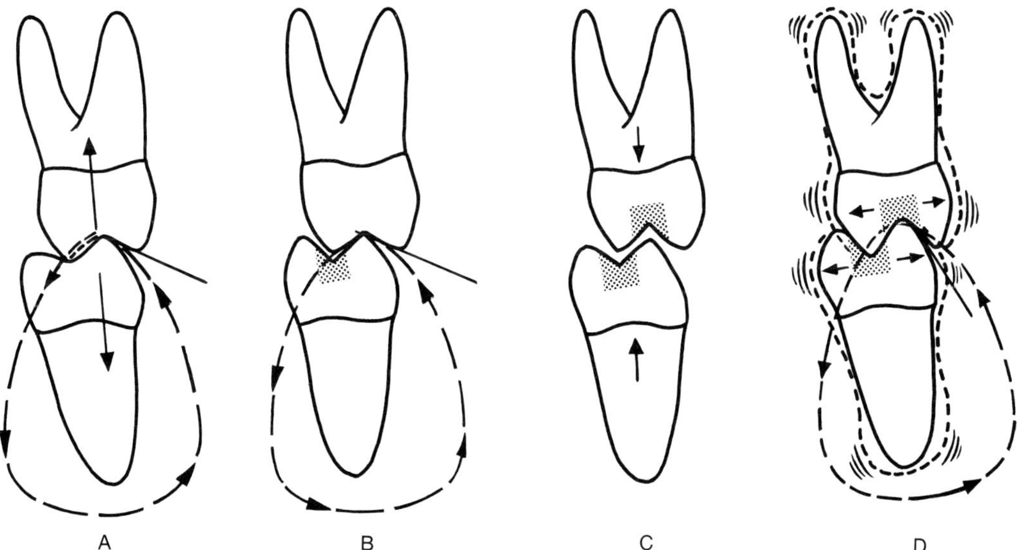

FIG. 58. **A,** Before restorations, teeth are axially loaded, (*arrows*) and there is lateral freedom. **B,** Restoration in lower tooth is overcarved. Upper lingual cusp does not contact restoration. Contact between lower cusp and upper fossa prevents extrusion, though tipping is possible. **C,** Restoration in upper tooth is overcarved. Lower cusp does not contact upper restoration. All occlusal contact has been eliminated, and eruption occurs (*arrows*). **D,** Teeth erupt into opposing occlusal surfaces, and lateral freedom is lost. Restraint occurs and patient now unconsciously bruxes.

As teeth erupt or (and) restorations wear or fracture, excursive interferences occur. The articulation of the teeth becomes more restrained as the cusps lock deeper into the opposing occlusal surfaces. Figure 58D shows the restrained angle of lateral movement the teeth now permit. This angle, which is now the same as the cuspal inclines, interferes with the normal and customary envelope of motion. Though the patient is not conscious of the restraint, the neuromuscular system feels it and the patient bruxes. The teeth are luxated horizontally. The result is severe occlusal traumatism, even though the MICP contact may produce axial loading.

RECAPITULATION

When Is the Lateral Adjustment Completed, or When Is a Lateral Pathway Created?

A lateral pathway is created when the marks on the working side consist of dots of MICP contact plus lines of lateral contact only on the index teeth. The lines on the index teeth are on as smooth a surface as possible.

The smooth plane of the index extends distal to the line of contact. Most of the time the lateral movement the patient makes is a protrusive lateral one. The freedom distally allows the patient to go to the border movement without any interference.

How Does One Know When the Line of Lateral Contact on the Index Tooth Is at a Reasonable Angle?

The line of lateral contact is at a reasonable angle when the mark is on the marginal ridge of the index tooth or is on a plane whose angle is the same as that of the marginal ridge of the index tooth. Naturally, the index tooth should be normally inclined in its position.

Why Is the Lateral-Pathway Concept Beneficial?

The lateral-pathway concept is beneficial because the only contact possible during lateral movement is on the index, which is a smooth surface. This establishment of a lateral pathway makes lateral tooth contacts impossible, except on the index tooth. It creates a situation of maximum freedom for mandibular motion and the best chance for *no contact* of the teeth during lateral movement. Even contact on the index tooth will be minimal.

What Are the Three Major Steps in Creating a Lateral Pathway?

(1) Elimination of the nonworking-side interferences, (2) creation of the index on the index teeth, and (3) elimination of lateral (working-side) interferences.

How Are Lateral Interferences Eliminated?

Select and adjust the index teeth. Then grind all marks representing lateral contact from all the teeth until only the index teeth contact during lateral motion. Make sure that marks of lateral contact on the index teeth are straight. These lines should be on as smooth a surface as possible. Make sure that the angle of these lines is correct. (More is said about checking this angle on pp. 79–81.)

How Long Does it Take to Create a Lateral Pathway?

After a little practice, the procedure can be done in a matter of minutes.

What if the Index Tooth Will Not Mark Along Its Marginal Ridge Area, and Instead the Mark from the Articulating Ribbon Is on the Cuspal Incline of the Cusp?

Grind the cuspal incline until the plane of the cuspal incline is the same as that of the marginal ridge.

Does that Not Mean a Lot of Grinding? Will the Tooth Not Become Sensitive?

No. Consider the grinding caused by bruxing. If the teeth survive long enough, the patient grinds not only the nonsupporting cusps (the buccal cusps of the upper teeth and the lingual cusps of the lower teeth) but also the supporting cusps (the buccal cusps of the lower teeth and the lingual cusps of the upper teeth). People brux to rid themselves of restraint, but they do not succeed. They are unable to change the angle of jaw motion by bruxing until they have worn the teeth in half. By this time they have probably lost most of their teeth. The remaining teeth are in danger or are liable to fracture. These people would be wiser to have a knowledgeable dentist grind their teeth rather than trying to do the job themselves. The dentist can rid them of restraint with a minimum of grinding, and he can do all the grinding on the correct teeth with a grinding stone. If the dentist does not grind, the patients must use their own teeth to grind with, and this compounds the problem. Of course, there is a point at which occlusal adjustment by selective grinding must give way to reconstruction or orthodontics. But grinding is the mainstay of occlusal treatment.

Can Occlusal Adjustment Stop Most Bruxing?

Yes. But there are some people who brux their teeth no matter what the dentist does. For these people it is necessary to construct a bite guard.

How Can One Justify the Statement that Occlusal Adjustment or the Creation of Freedom in an Occlusion Can Stop Bruxing?

The clinical experience of many dentists has shown this to be true, but you can easily prove the truth of this to yourself. The next time you are going to place a posterior restoration into occlusion, place a temporary restoration first. Place the cement and have the patient bite into it so that it is not high in the MICP. Do not take away any cement so as to create lateral freedom. Trim the excess but leave a definite imprint of the opposing cusp tip in the cement (Fig. 57). Tell the patient he may go, but observe him carefully. He may not let you get away with what you have done. He may tell you something is wrong. He will start bruxing the cement immediately. If the patient thinks you cannot make a mistake, he may leave the office. If he does, observe him without his seeing you. Watch what he does. You will notice a strained expression on his face and that he is making bruxing movements.

As soon as you are satisfied that bruxing can be induced immediately, have mercy on the patient and adjust the temporary restoration. Give the filling freedom by relieving the inclines until the only contact the patient can make on the filling is a pinpoint contact in the MICP.

As soon as you have adjusted the cement correctly, the patient's face will begin to look calmer and more relaxed. He will stop bruxing. (If you really want to get the feel of this experiment, have someone do it on you.)

Different people react differently to restraint. Some patients go home and try to live with it. Some refuse to leave the office until the filling is properly adjusted.

Emotions determine to a great extent what people do with their teeth. Calm people can have interferences that to them are not interferences since they do not cause them to brux. However, tense people with the same occlusal design may brux their teeth until they become loosened or worn.

Since dentists cannot evaluate the emotional makeup of each patient, establish a lateral pathway that permits maximum freedom. This will allow people who brux to stop bruxing. Remember that bruxism is caused by tension and that, depending on your occlusal adjustment, you can create or relieve tension in your patients.

How Does One Know When There Is Freedom of Lateral Motion and No Restraint of Lateral Motion?

There is no specific angle that can be said to be correct. The angle of a lateral pathway that works is correct. When it works, the patient does not bother to brux the index tooth.

We suggest that, to achieve this state, you use the marginal-ridge angle of a normally inclined index tooth as the criterion for establishing the angle of a lateral pathway. This approach is reasonable, but you can check still further by testing for fremitus.

FREMITUS

Fremitus is a most important clinical test for early occlusal traumatism. When present, fremitus indicates that a tooth is receiving horizontal forces and that changes in the bony housing of the tooth have begun to take place, but are not yet sufficient to have produced mobility or further damage. Determining the presence of fremitus and eliminating it are skills necessary for the treatment and prevention of occlusal traumatism.

Fremitus is a slight movement or vibration in an upper tooth that the dentist can feel with his finger when the patient rubs or taps his teeth together. To check for fremitus of the index tooth, place the tip of your finger on the facial surface of the index tooth near the gingival margin. Have the patient make a lateral bruxing movement toward the side where your finger is (the working side). If you have made a good, smooth index, you will not be able to feel any fremitus of the upper tooth during the lateral movement (Fig. 59). Also, the patient will be able to make the movement easily upon your command.

Each time the patient returns for recall appointments, check the index tooth. Check to make sure (1) it is firm (there is no fremitus) and (2) it is free of continued wear. Since the index tooth is the only tooth that contacts during lateral movement, chances are that you have eliminated bruxing when it shows neither fremitus nor wear. If the index tooth shows fremitus,

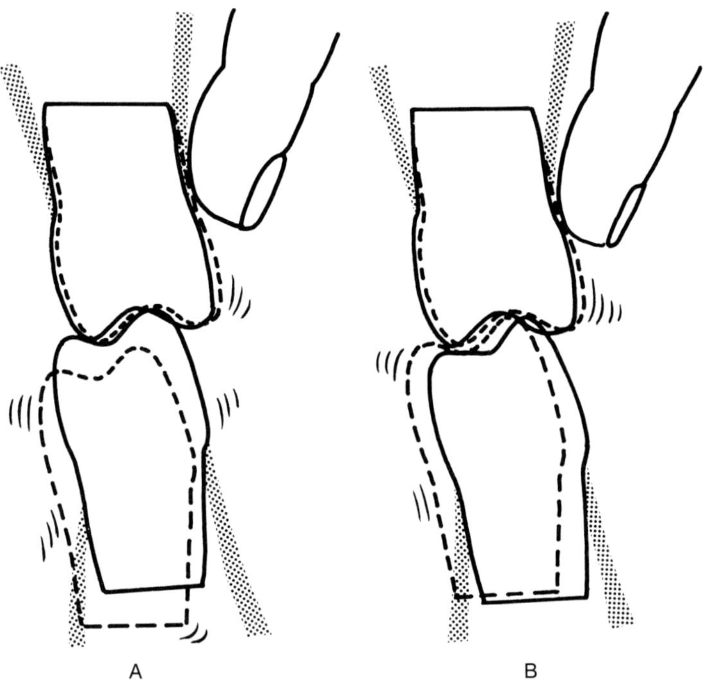

A   B

FIG. 59. To check for fremitus, hold finger very lightly at junction of gingiva and tooth. Finger should be partly on gingiva and partly on tooth. **A,** To check for fremitus in MICP, have patient rapidly tap teeth firmly together a number of times. Any vibration of tooth is fremitus. **B,** To check for fremitus during lateral movement, have patient rub teeth against each other from side to side. Any vibration of tooth is fremitus. Vibrations can be felt better if finger is on more than one tooth at a time.

‚mobility, or wear, with the following in mind double-check your adjustment.

1. The angle of the index may still be too steep for the particular patient. Reduce the angle of the index; make it more horizontal.

2. The lateral index may be rough rather than glass smooth. Make it smooth.

3. There may be a rough or ditched area on another tooth making contact during the initial instant of lateral motion. Find it and eliminate it to the point at which there is only a pinpoint MICP contact.

4. There may be a nonworking-side interference. Eliminate it.

5. If everything checks out and the patient appears to be a compulsive bruxer, make him a bite guard. Training patients in muscle-relaxation skills is also a promising new area of dental treatment.

The ideal lateral pathway allows so much freedom that the patient does not hit the index tooth. If lateral or eccentric tooth contact is not made, the patient cannot traumatize his teeth. In other words, if the index allows for extreme lateral movement, there will be adequate freedom from restraint and the patient will usually not care to make lateral bruxing movements.

Remember, however, that there are occlusal factors other than lateral restraint that can cause bruxing. They are:

1. A contact dot in the MICP that is too wide buccolingually (pp. 64, 65, 121, 122)

2. A lack of holding boundaries, resulting in a loss of stability (pp. 9, 10)

3. Protrusive restraint (pp. 89–100)

4. Restraint to centric relation (pp. 10–13)

When a complete occlusal adjustment has been done, you can then check the index tooth. As long as it does not show fremitus, mobility, or new wear, you can assume that the patient is not habitually bruxing. The occlusal adjustment is successful.

CLASS I AND CLASS II OCCLUSIONS

The problem of the Class II occlusion was briefly discussed on page 54. Let us now take a deeper look at it (Fig. 60).

In the Class I occlusion, the lower cusp enters and leaves the mesial fossae of the upper teeth. The upper buccal cusps are not in the path of lateral movement on either the working or non-working side, nor do they restrain protrusive movement.

In the Class II occlusion, the lower buccal cusps enter and leave the distal fossae of the upper teeth. The upper buccal cusps are interfering with the path of lateral movement of the lower cusps on both the working and nonworking sides as well as restraining protrusive movement.

Note that the cuspid and bicuspid interfere with lateral movements more than do the molars in the Class II occlusion. Because of the curvature of the arch, there is a greater protrusive component to lateral movement in the cuspid and bicuspid areas of the dental arch.

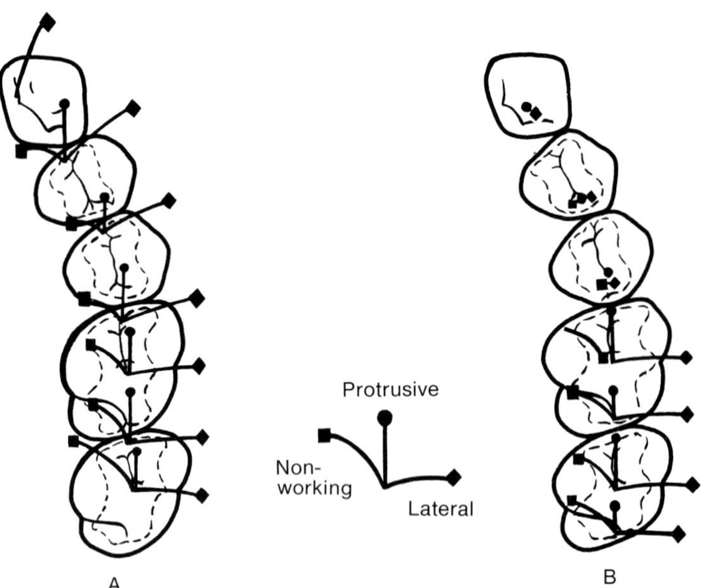

FIG. 60. *A,* Class I occlusion allows greater freedom for all jaw movements. *B,* Class II occlusion restrains all mandibular movements; lateral, nonworking-side, and protrusive.

ANOTHER LOOK AT THE LATERAL INDEX

The lateral index, like an incisal guide table, provides for the creation of a lateral pathway. We speak of certain teeth touching during lateral movement and we design these contacts at a particular angle. It may sound as if eccentric or lateral tooth contacts are designed as functional contacts. Yet we have also said that the best eccentric occlusal contact is no contact at all. In other words, are we going to a lot of trouble to develop occlusal anatomy (lateral pathways) so that the teeth will *not* touch in eccentric positions?

The term *lateral index* is used because it represents a way of thinking. Some may ask why the term *guidance* is not used. The reason it is not used is that, in relation to occlusion, *guidance* means different things to different dentists. It represents too many ways of thinking. There exist lateral guidance, cuspid guidance, incisal guidance, group function occlusion, mutually protected occlusion, fully balanced occlusion, and so on.

To produce any of the above-mentioned occlusal schemes, it is true that the mandible must be guided. No matter what the articulators or dental instruments in use today, there is an element of guidance that must be provided empirically in order to develop an occlusal scheme.

Dentists can make accurate pantographs, locate centers of rotation, make functionally generated paths and know they are correct for the individual patient. But, rather empirically, the incisal guide or its equivalent must be set on the articulator and adjusted on the teeth in the mouth; or the incisal guidance the patient already has must be accepted or modified. How to do this causes much discussion in dentistry.

The technique of each occlusal scheme dictates how to determine this guidance, because until it has been determined it is impossible to carve the occlusal anatomy of the teeth. The descriptions of how to determine it are excellent and they provide good results, but it must be realized that no two dentists would arrive at an exactly identical guidance for a particular patient. There would be a closeness but not an exactness.

Getting to the point of exactness is really no problem because exactness is an impossible ideal. There is no exact guidance. Attempting exactness is self-defeating. The problem is how to set the incisal guide or its equivalent to achieve the objective —freedom of lateral movement.

A method of thinking and arriving at your own solutions to the problem can be found in the concept of the lateral index. The term *lateral index* is not associated with any technique for extensive prosthesis. And a concept is needed to apply to the young occlusion that provides a way of thinking about routine dentistry that is done on the relatively healthy dentition. The disease is already advanced when all the teeth have to be prepared, the case mounted on an adjustable articulator, and then the incisal guide table set. When the disease arrives at this late stage, there is no problem getting ourselves to think about setting the incisal guide table on the articulator. However, dentistry should set the incisal guide at an early age, before severe occlusal disease destroys the mouth.

The lateral index should be thought of in terms of prevention as well as of treatment; it is offered to stimulate more preventive occlusal treatment. It can be used for occlusal adjustment of the natural dentition by selective grinding before the reconstruction is necessary. The lateral index could be used restoration by restoration to build resistant preventive occlusal anatomy. The concept can be used during orthodontic treatment so that collapse of the occlusion does not occur.

Dentists would agree that this is a good idea. But some might still object to a new term. They might argue that an acceptable guidance can be established for a particular patient and carried through with all subsequent restorations and dental work.

Just as *lateral index* represents a way of thinking, so does *guidance*. To some, guidance means that all mandibular movement is guided by the teeth. This idea is projected further until the dentist feels that he determines or guides the mandibular movement of his patients—a dangerous way of thinking.

True, the teeth do guide mandibular movement, and the dentist by modifying teeth can enter into or participate in guiding mandibular movement. However, the question is, to what degree should the teeth guide mandibular movement? The answer is, to the degree that the *patient* will tolerate such guidance and to the degree that the patient's neuromuscular makeup will accept and move the mandible within the confines of the tooth guidance.

The important point is that the teeth can guide mandibular movement only with the consent of the patient, i.e., with the consent of his neuromuscular makeup. When the patient consents to tooth guidance, he no longer uses tooth guidance. To state this another way: Once the patient learns where the occlusal anatomy is and accepts it, he consents to move the mandible within the boundaries of the occlusal anatomy without hitting these boundaries or making nonfunctional lateral tooth contacts, such as bruxing.

If the patient uses the tooth guidance continuously, the teeth are guiding mandibular movement. Or would it not be wiser to say that the teeth are restraining mandibular movement rather than guiding it? This is why the patient keeps grinding his teeth. The teeth in this case are not guiding the mandible by consent of the patient, but rather restraining the mandible in spite of the patient.

When the teeth spite the patient, the teeth usually suffer. The patient's neuromuscular system will knock the teeth out or wear the interfering occlusal anatomy away, or do both.

Some might say that not all bruxism results from occlusal anatomy interfering with mandibular motion, that we do not know why some people brux. True. We agree with these observations. The lack of knowledge indicates that we cannot cure psychological problems by occlusal treatment. Nevertheless, we can help the vast majority of people with occlusal problems.

Again, the point to be made here is that tooth guidance, if it is acceptable, for the most part does not guide a thing. The mandible should be free to be guided by the patient's neuromuscular makeup within the boundaries of the occlusal anatomy. If the neuromuscular makeup accepts the occlusal anatomy, the neuromuscular system learns to move the mandible within the boundaries of the occlusal anatomy and the mandible rarely bumps into those boundaries

Thus successful lateral guidance, cuspid guidance, incisal guidance, along with the various eccentric occlusal schemes, such as group function, mutually protected occlusion, fully balanced occlusion, and so on are successful only when learned and accepted by the patient, not when used by the patient.

Since dentists are not routinely using fully adjustable articulators for occlusal adjustment by selective grinding or for routine restorations and bridgework, they must have a practical way to establish an acceptable lateral pathway. They need guidelines; they need to know (1) which teeth to build the lateral index on and (2) at what angle to build the lateral pathway. The lateral index gives a start toward acceptability and consistency among dentists.

The Plane of the Lateral Index Is Parallel to the Plane of the Marginal Ridges

All schools of occlusion recommend cusp pass-thru for lateral movement and that the lower cusp path be on the upper marginal ridges or in grooves that are on planes parallel to that of the marginal ridges. The reason is that if the cusp tip goes on the steeper angle of the cuspal incline of the opposing cusp, there is restraint of normal muscle action.

Therefore, to prevent restraint in lateral movement, the patient should move laterally either on the marginal ridges or on a plane that is parallel to that of the marginal ridges. In reconstruction this is not a major problem because the cusp tips can be placed right on the marginal ridges. However, most operative dentistry consists of placing amalgams or, at most, a few restorations. Therefore, the dentist has to work with the intercuspation the patient presents, and most of the time the cusp tip moves excursively on the cuspal inclines.

When this condition exists, in order to establish lateral freedom, that part of the cuspal incline that is contacted by the opposing cusp tip is ground so that the plane of contact is parallel to the plane of the marginal ridge. Now, when the patient makes a lateral movement, instead of being forced out at the steep angle of the cuspal incline he will be moving at the same angle as if he were on the marginal ridge.

Wear and Cusp Tips

The less the teeth touch, the less aware the person is of his occlusion. The less a person is aware of his occlusion, consciously or unconsciously, the less he grinds, bruxes, or clenches his teeth. The less the teeth touch, the less the occlusal trauma and tooth wear.

However, teeth do touch and teeth do wear. Occasionally, patients do clench or brux their teeth, and the cusp tips do touch during swallowing. Does the cusp tip wear disproportionately compared to the cusp seat or index?

Diets in civilization cause relatively little wear. Most wear is due to bruxing. Since freedom stops most bruxing, it will stop most cusp-tip wear. However, even if a patient were to contact his index occasionally, the wear of the cusp tip would not be extensive.

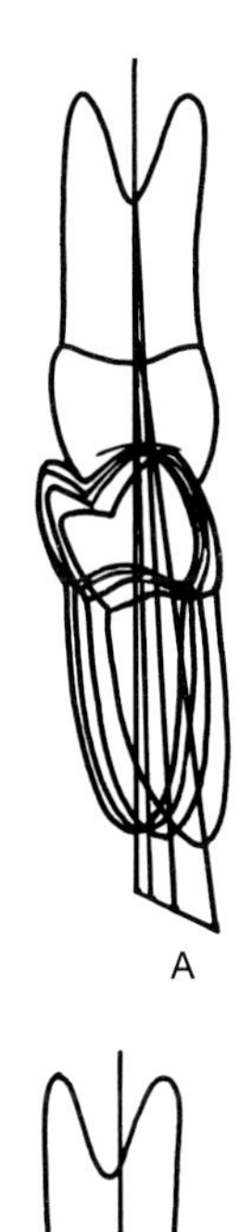

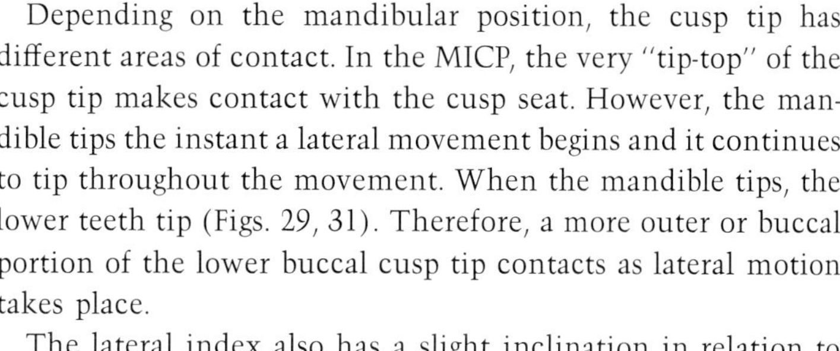

Depending on the mandibular position, the cusp tip has different areas of contact. In the MICP, the very "tip-top" of the cusp tip makes contact with the cusp seat. However, the mandible tips the instant a lateral movement begins and it continues to tip throughout the movement. When the mandible tips, the lower teeth tip (Figs. 29, 31). Therefore, a more outer or buccal portion of the lower buccal cusp tip contacts as lateral motion takes place.

The lateral index also has a slight inclination in relation to the cusp seat. This additionally results in the lower buccal cusp tip making contact farther down its buccal incline.

Only the Lower Buccal Cusp Remains In Contact During a Lateral Bruxing Jaw Movement

The same tipping of the mandibular tooth that moves lateral contact from the tip of the cusp to its buccal surface also tends to drop the lower lingual cusp out of contact with its opposing upper lingual cusp (Fig. 61). Therefore, when a posterior tooth is used as an index tooth, the only contact during a lateral jaw movement is between the lower buccal cusp and the upper lateral index.

A Last Word about Lateral Adjustment

In regard to doing a complete occlusal adjustment by selective grinding, we do not recommend excursive adjustment before centric relation; but for learning purposes, we do suggest practicing occlusal adjustment in this fashion and order.

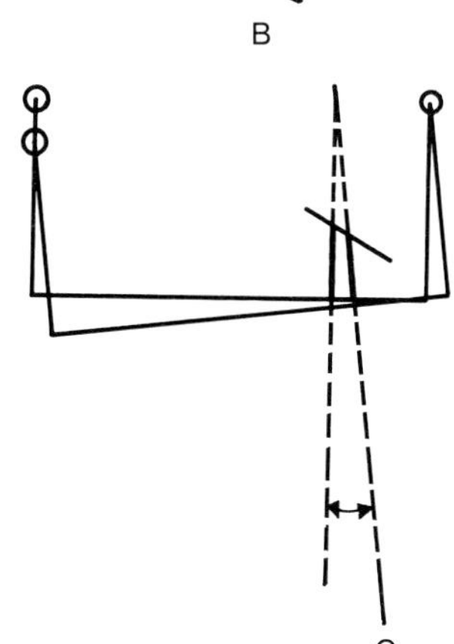

FIG. 61. During lateral movement, lingual half of lower tooth tips away from upper lingual cusp. **A,** As lower tooth moves buccally, it tips. Note changes in axial inclination relative to upper tooth. This, plus inclination of lateral pathway, tips the lower lingual cusp away from upper lingual cusp and moves contact of lower buccal cusp from tip to area just buccal to cusp tip. **B,** Tipping of lower tooth with resultant changed axial inclination relative to upper tooth. **C,** Nonworking-side condyle orbits around working-side condyle. This results in tipping of mandible during lateral motion. Because mandible tips, lower teeth tip, and, therefore, lower lingual cusps tip away from upper lingual cusps.

FOR SELF-EVALUATION

1. What is the ideal in regard to lateral contact?

2. Once the MICP contact has been established, what is a most important rule during the adjustment of lateral?

3. Where, on an upper tooth, will nonworking-side contacts occur most often?

4. To relieve nonworking-side contact, is most of the grinding usually done on an upper or on a lower tooth?

5. What is the lateral index?

6. What is the index tooth?

7. We prefer the cuspid, or the most anterior of the posterior teeth, as the index tooth. What are the three most important criteria for choosing an index tooth?

8. After the lateral index is adjusted, how is the lateral pathway made?

9. What is the most common and damaging error in relieving the excursive contacts from the posterior teeth?

10. What is lateral freedom?

11. Why is lateral freedom important?

12. What natural anatomic landmark on a tooth helps in determining lateral freedom?

13. What are the three major steps in creating a lateral pathway?

4

Providing Protrusive Freedom

(The Protrusive Pathway) on Posterior Teeth

PROTRUSIVE CONTACTS ON POSTERIOR TEETH

When the posterior teeth are in contact during a protrusive movement, we apply the same principles of freedom from restraint as were applied to lateral movements. First, the most anterior of the posterior teeth should be the only ones contacted during a protrusive movement. Second, the protrusive glide should be glass smooth. Third, the protrusive glide should be controlled by the neuromuscular system and not interfered with or restrained by cuspal inclines.

It is important that, if at all possible, molars do not contact during a protrusive movement (Fig. 62). Protrusive contact should be allowed only on bicuspids. While it is best to have the protrusive glide as horizontal as possible, because the glide takes place on the holding boundaries of the bicuspids and you must not lose your holding boundaries, there is not much flattening that can be done. Usually, however, there is not much that needs to be done. It is important that the protrusive glide be made smooth.

Because of the coordination of the temporomandibular joints and bilateral muscle symmetry, the neuromuscular system moves the mandible straight forward during a protrusive jaw movement. Any cuspal restraint will cause the mandible to deviate to one side or the other. It is important to relieve all

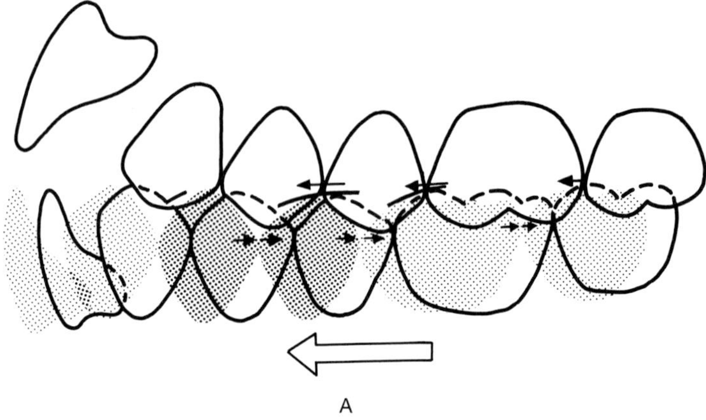

A

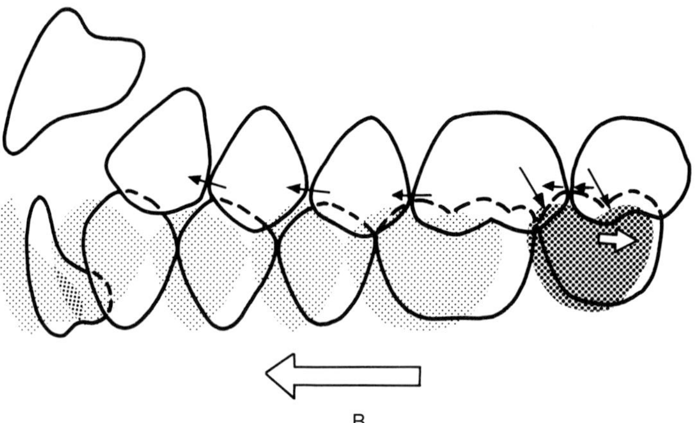

B

FIG. 62. **A,** Correct distribution of protrusive contacts on posterior teeth during protrusive glide. Only bicuspids contact, and protrusive movement is smooth and straight forward. Distal force on bicuspids (*arrows at contact points of lower teeth*) is taken up by more posterior teeth, and all teeth remain stable. Arrows in upper teeth indicate protusive pathway. **B,** Incorrect distribution of protrusive contacts on posterior teeth during protrusive movement. Vertical arrows indicate protrusive contact on lower second molar. This drives lower second molar distally (*white arrow*) and opens contact between it and first molar.

such interferences and allow the neuromuscular system to move the mandible straight forward under its control.

To achieve these objectives, we use the concept of the protrusive pathway.

THE PROTRUSIVE PATHWAY

The *protrusive pathway* is a space through which the lower cusps pass during protrusive and retrusive jaw movement. As with the lateral pathway, the protrusive pathway is designed so that tooth contact during protrusive motion is unlikely. This is in agreement with our concept of preventing as much excursive tooth contact as possible.

The protrusive pathway must allow for an undeflected forward movement of the mandible. The mandible should not have to deviate to the right or left to get around an interfering tooth surface.

Technique

The protrusive pathway is created by the systematic removal of protrusive interferences.

I. Select the index teeth for the protrusive adjustment. Use tight upper bicuspids on each side that have contact in the MICP (Fig. 62). (Naturally, the upper cuspids are the preferred protrusive index teeth, but we are discussing a situation in which the anterior teeth are absent or out of occlusion. Protrusive adjustment of the anterior teeth will be discussed later.)

    Do not use molars as protrusive index teeth if more anterior teeth are available. The force on a lower molar in protrusive contact is in a distal direction. The force on the upper tooth is mesial in direction. Thus all the teeth mesial to the upper tooth (assuming proximal contact) help support it, but the lower last molar with no tooth distal can be separated from its mesial neighbor. Besides the trauma from occlusion on the lower molar, the open contact leads to food impaction, which further insults the periodontium (Fig. 62).

II. Mark the teeth during a protrusive movement. To do this, dry the teeth and place articulating ribbon between the posterior teeth. Ask the patient to close in the MICP and then rub the teeth together during a straight forward protrusive movement of the jaw. The patient may need your assistance in this maneuver in order to avoid deviation of the mandible to one side or the other. Let him hold a hand mirror and watch his own movement.

If anterior teeth are present, make a vertical line on the upper anterior teeth coinciding with the midline of the lower incisors. Make this mark while the teeth are held together in the MICP.

If the upper and lower arch midlines are coincidental, no mark is necessary. Just ask the patient to move his jaw protrusively while keeping the midlines in line or opposite each other.

III. Grind away all marks made by the protrusive motion on all the teeth except the index teeth. *Do not grind away any MICP contacts during the protrusive adjustment.*

IV. Adjust the markings on the index teeth until they are smooth. Do this by making the area smooth between the MICP contact and the end of the protrusive marking.

V. Check the results by re-marking the teeth during the protrusive movement. If marks from the protrusive movement occur on any teeth other than the index teeth, remove them.

The result of the protrusive adjustment will be a dot on the tip of a lower buccal cusp and a line on the distal inner slopes of the upper protrusive index teeth.

MORE ABOUT PROTRUSIVE INTERFERENCE

Where Do Protrusive Interferences Appear?

Protrusive interferences appear on the mesial inner slopes of lower lingual cusps and the distal inner slopes of upper buccal cusps.

How Are Protrusive Interferences Adjusted?

Grind away all protrusive marks until only the index teeth mark during a protrusive movement. Grind the area between the MICP mark and the end of the most medial portion of the protrusive mark flat and smooth.

When we speak of grinding the lateral or protrusive index on an index tooth flat and smooth, we do not mean that the cusps are ground off so that they are flattened. We mean that the line of contact of the lower cusp tip on the upper tooth should not have a wavy or bumpy surface. In other words, the line of contact on the surface of the tooth is made flat even though it is on an incline. Then the surface is made smooth by polishing it.

Then What?

Re-mark the teeth during protrusive motion and check to make sure that only the index teeth have protrusive markings.

What Do the Protrusive Marks Finally Look Like on the Index Teeth?

Assuming the use of red articulating ribbon, the marks look like straight red lines on smooth distal inner slopes of upper buccal cusps and (or) marginal ridges. These marks have been made by the tips of the opposing lower buccal cusps.

Are There Corresponding Lines or Protrusive Markings on the Mesial Inner Slopes of Lower Lingual Cusps?

No. Excursive markings appear only on index teeth and only upper teeth are index teeth. (In a crossbite occlusion the index teeth may be lower teeth.)

FOR SELF-EVALUATION

1. What is meant by protrusive restraint?

2. In normally related teeth, which cuspal inclines cause protrusive interferences?

3. Which posterior teeth are the best to use as protrusive index teeth? Why?

5

Establishing Occlusion on the Anterior Teeth

It is not desirable therapeutically that the anterior teeth contact in the MICP, because in the MICP the muscles can exert tremendous force. This force can be directed axially on posterior teeth but *not* on anterior teeth. Therefore, to effect anterior tooth contact in the MICP would be violating a basic principle of occlusion, namely the principle of axial forces. The cusp seat axially loads the posterior teeth, and its holding boundary can maintain a positive and stable MICP that prevents the anterior teeth from contacting.

One need not worry about the lower anterior teeth erupting into contact. When the anterior teeth are properly adjusted, they just miss contacting each other—by a hair's breadth. Feather-light excursive contacts and normal grasping and incising of food will prevent the lower anterior teeth from extruding into MICP contact.

FEATHER-LIGHT INCISOR CONTACT IN EXCURSIVE MOTION

The anterior teeth can make light excursive contacts with each other, but the cuspid is the preferred predominant contact (Fig. 63). The lateral protrusive indices on the cuspids are definite clear marks of contact. Remember, however, that these marks can be made only by having the patient brux. If the indices are made at acceptable angles, the patient is unlikely to strike them during function.

Maintenance of Feather-Light Occlusal Contacts and Tooth Positions

There are four safety factors involved in maintaining feather-light occlusal contacts and tooth relationships.

1.   The anterior teeth are used in grasping and incising. This type of function axially loads the anterior teeth. When one bites into an apple, for instance, the apple is placed between the anterior teeth and pushed posteriorly as the bite is made. This is an axial force, and a fairly light force, which is not going to be traumatic to the normal dentition.

2.   Muscle power is reduced the instant the jaw moves out of the MICP. Excursive movement requires a balance between the protagonist and antagonist muscles, so that it is impossible to exert as much force on the teeth during excursive movement as it is in the MICP. Place your hands on the side of your face, covering the masseter and temporal muscles. Squeeze your teeth together tightly and feel how these muscles flex and bulge; while the muscles are flexed, begin to move your jaw in any excursive motion. You will note that the masseter and temporal muscles relax somewhat as the external pterygoid muscle begins to contract and balance against the other two. This automatically reduces the power potential on the teeth in excursive movement.

3.   The smaller the angle of contact in relation to the horizon, the less the force that can be applied on the teeth. Also, the smaller the angle, the less the chance for one to rub his teeth together; he will grasp and incise with them only.

4.   The farther the teeth are positioned away from the fulcrum in a second-class lever mechanism, the less the power that can be exerted. The anterior teeth are the farthest from the fulcrum, the temporomandibular joint.

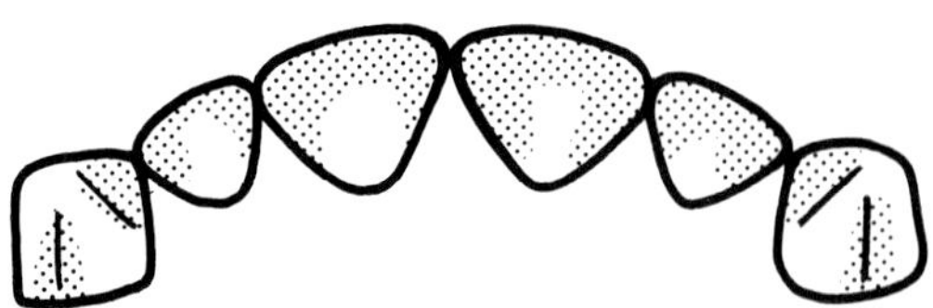

FIG. 63. Desired occlusal markings on lingual surfaces of upper anterior teeth. Vertical lines on distal of cuspids are protrusive indices. Diagonal lines on mesial of cuspids are lateral indices. Shaded areas represent brush contacts of incisors during lateral and protrusive movement. Brush contact marks are light and indefinite smudges. Lateral and protrusive indices are definite heavy marks of contact.

TECHNIQUE FOR ADJUSTING ANTERIOR TEETH

I. **ADJUST THE OVERBITE CONTACT IF PRESENT.** When there is a deep overbite with a facet on the labial surface of the lower anterior teeth and on the lingual surface of the upper anterior teeth, reduce the overbite. This is done by grinding the incisal edges of the upper and lower anterior teeth until the desired overbite is established. (Figs. 64, 65A, B).

One might ask, what is desired? What is a normal overbite? There are no exact answers. You must be guided to a large extent by the averages and by the anatomy of the teeth. We would certainly think twice about grinding into the pulp just to establish a "normal" overbite. Two millimeters is permissible. So are three and four millimeters if the teeth are well adjusted or aligned. Try to avoid extremes and to correct existing ones.

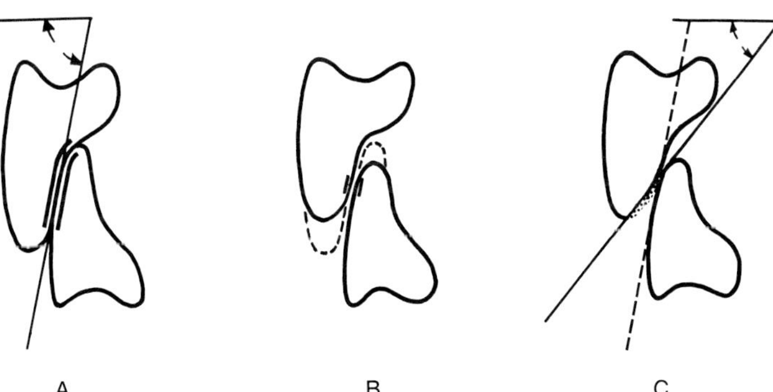

A   B   C

FIG. 64. *A,* Deep overbite relationship. Heavy lines represent areas of MICP contact. Thin line passing between heavy lines represents angle of contact in relation to horizontal plane. This is angle of protrusive movement dictated by teeth. *B,* Amount of grinding done on incisal edges of teeth to reduce overbite. Dotted outline shows original shape of teeth. MICP contact is reduced, as illustrated by short, heavy black lines. *C,* Amount ground from lingual surface of upper tooth to permit acceptable lateral and protrusive movements (freedom). Portion ground away is shaded. Grinding reduces MICP contact to pinpoint size, or to thin line if viewed from front. Thin line passing between dots shows angle now permitted for protrusive movement in relation to horizontal plane. Dashed line shows original angle of protrusive movement.

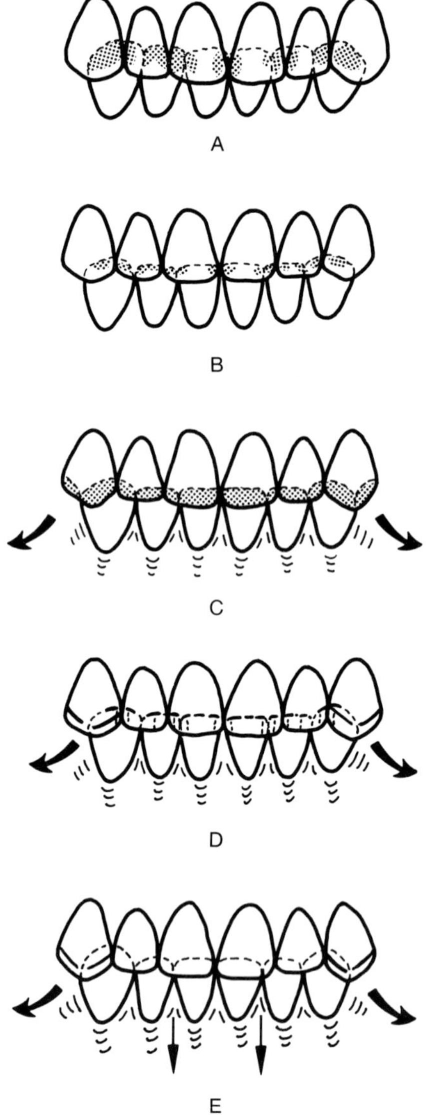

FIG. 65. The anterior adjustment. **A,** Deep overbite from frontal view. Contact between teeth is shaded. **B,** Reduction of overbite by grinding incisal edges of teeth. Reduced contact areas shaded. **C,** Contact areas during lateral protrusive movement illustrated by shaded portions. **D,** Lateral contacts adjusted (contact areas of **C** adjusted). Dark horizontal lines are MICP contacts. Lateral indices on cuspids shown as angled lines on mesial of cuspids. Protrusive indices made by lower first bicuspids (not shown) are angled lines on distal of cuspids. Vertical dotted lines on incisors indicate protrusive index on incisors if impossible to make lower first bicuspids contact upper cuspids during protrusive glide. **E,** Final step in adjustment is removal of MICP contacts from lingual of upper anterior teeth.

Large facets on the labial surfaces of the lower anterior teeth and the lingual surfaces of the upper anterior teeth suggest that improvement can be made. Try to decrease the overbite by grinding the incisal edges of the upper and lower anterior teeth. Let esthetics help decide whether you should take more off the upper anterior teeth or more off the lower anterior teeth. Have the patient smile. If too much upper tooth shows, grind the incisal edges of the upper teeth; if it does not, grind the lower incisal edges. Use judgment. You may wish to remove some from both the upper and the lower teeth.

Whatever teeth are ground, be sure that the grinding is done on their incisal edges. Do not grind the labial aspect of the lower anterior teeth. Do not eliminate the MICP contact from between the anterior teeth at this time.

II. **ADJUST THE MICP CONTACT IF IT IS STILL IN THE FORM OF A FACET.** Have the patient tap the teeth together in the MICP with articulating ribbon between them. Grind away all of the smudges on the lingual surfaces of the upper anterior teeth *except* the most apical line or mark of contact.

Check the results of this step by repeating it. As a result of this adjustment, the MICP contact should be seen as a horizontal line or dot on the lingual surfaces of the upper anterior teeth and on the incisal edges of the lower anterior teeth. The marks should be sharp and definite, not large smudges.

In the young dentition, there may not be any facet or smudge-like contact between the anterior teeth. The MICP contacts may already be satisfactory. If so, the adjustment of the anterior teeth begins with Step III.

If the MICP contacts are already sharp, definite dots or lines, a deep overbite can be adjusted only by grinding the incisal edges of the upper anterior teeth.

III. **ADJUST THE INCISORS TO FEATHER-LIGHT OR BRUSH CONTACT.** Grind the marks on the lingual surfaces of the upper incisors until the cuspid marks heavier than the incisors. Here we must assume that the cuspid is the index tooth and that it has already been adjusted as described on pages 62–64. If a posterior tooth is used as an index tooth, all the upper anterior teeth, including the cuspid, are ground until they mark lighter than the index tooth.

Naturally, if any tooth except the index tooth marks during lateral motion the mark should be adjusted until it is lighter or absent. Do *not* grind the teeth way out of excursive contact in relation to the index tooth. The index tooth can contact in excursive motion, and the rest of the teeth should almost contact or just miss each other (Fig. 65C).

IV.   **ADJUST THE ANGLE OF POSSIBLE PROTRUSIVE CONTACT.** Dry the anterior teeth and place articulating ribbon between them. Have the patient close in the MICP and rub the front teeth together in a protrusive movement. Guide the mandible straight forward so that there is no lateral deviation in the motion. To do this, place a vertical pencil line on the labial surfaces of the upper and lower incisor teeth at the midline if they do not coincide with each other in the MICP. Give the patient a hand mirror and have him move protrusively, keeping the lines directly opposite each other or the midlines directly opposite each other, whichever the case might be.

Adjust the marks by grinding on the lingual surfaces of the upper anterior teeth until the marks from protrusive motion are as even as possible. Next, polish on the marks of the upper incisors until the upper cuspids mark the heaviest (Fig. 65D).

Sometimes it is impossible to get the cuspids to contact in a protrusive movement. If this is the case, grind the lingual surfaces of the upper incisors until they mark as evenly as possible and until the angle of the protrusive movement is as small as possible in relation to the horizontal plane.

When anterior teeth contact in a protrusive movement, all protrusive contact should be eliminated from the posterior teeth. The only time this is not the case is when the incisors are mobile and unacceptable as protrusive index teeth; an upper bicuspid on each side then becomes a protrusive index tooth. In such a case, follow the instructions for adjusting protrusive contacts on posterior teeth (pp. 89–92).

V. **ELIMINATE THE MICP CONTACT ON THE ANTERIOR TEETH.**
The last step in an occlusal adjustment is the elimination of the contact between the anterior teeth in the MICP. To do this, dry the anterior teeth, place articulating ribbon between them, and have the patient tap the teeth together in the MICP. Polish away the marks on the lingual surfaces of all six upper anterior teeth (Fig. 65E).

Check the results. Hold cellophane between the anterior teeth and have the patient close in the MICP. Pull on the cellophane. You should be able to pull it from between the anterior teeth. If you cannot, repeat the procedure of marking and polishing until the cellophane is released from between the anterior teeth in the MICP.

A well-adjusted occlusion is one in which:

1.   The posterior cusp tips and fossae or cusp seats contact in the MICP

2.   No anterior teeth contact in the MICP

3.   Only the index teeth contact during excursive motion

4.   The rest of the teeth miss each other by a hair's breadth during excursive movement (Fig. 66.)

The Smile Line and Tooth Cosmetics

Changes in the incisal edges of the anterior teeth can dramatically improve a person's appearance. The key to anterior cosmetics is the smile line. Whenever you have a chance to improve the smile line of your patient's teeth, do it.

The smile line is the line assumed by the lower lip during smiling. For best cosmetics, the incisal edges of the upper anterior teeth should be adjusted so that they follow this line. Grind the incisal edges of the lateral incisors about .5 millimeters shorter than the central incisors. Round the mesial incisal edges slightly and the distal incisal edges more. Have the incisal embrasures get progressively deeper and wider from the central incisors to the first bicuspids.

Never tell a patient that you are going to make his teeth or smile attractive, a statement that would imply his smile is not

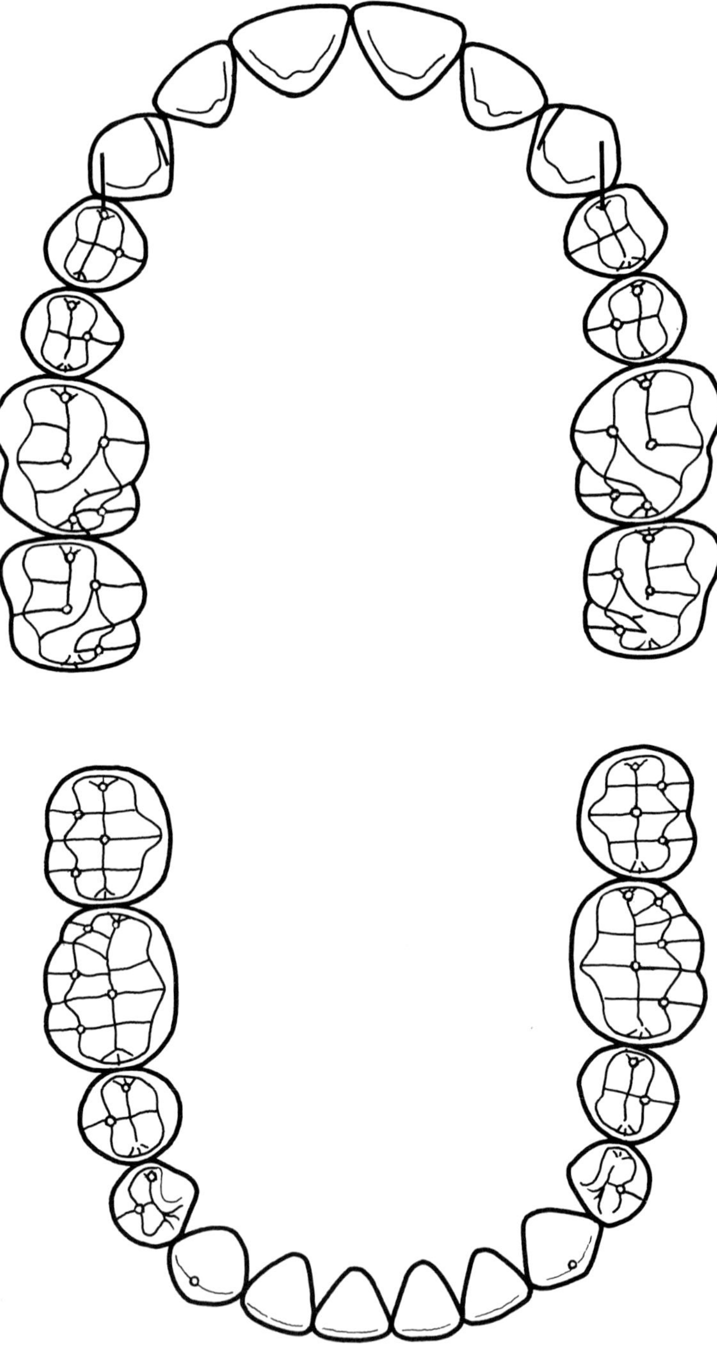

FIG. 66. You cannot make all, or even most, occlusal treatments ideal, as this one is. But you can, and should, create freedom from restraint, stability, and axial loading.

now attractive. Tell him you are going to make his teeth or smile *more* attractive as well as treat his bite and make it healthy.

THE COLD-SHOWER EFFECT

There is still another important reason for having the anterior teeth just out of contact in the MICP and making light or brush contact in excursive movements. We call the reason the cold-shower effect.

Suppose you step unaware from a warm room into a cold shower. Reflexly, without thinking, you jump out. Why? Change. The human body reflexly avoids abrupt change.

Now suppose that as you went into the cold shower someone slammed the shower door so that you could not get out. In a short time you would get used to the cold water if the temperature was within reason. It would no longer feel so cold.

The same principle applies to the teeth. Suppose that the anterior teeth do not touch in the MICP. Imagine placing a crown that makes one of them touch. Would the patient tell you it is high? Indeed he would. He would insist that you grind it until it feels the way it used to feel.

But suppose that you tell the patient that the crown is supposed to touch a little. Although he is not too sure you are right, he accepts the explanation and leaves the office. Within a few days he adjusts to the change and does not notice the contact any more. Even if the tooth becomes loose, the patient will usually not be aware of it.

When the anterior teeth do not touch in the MICP and do touch in excursive movement, the patient tends to get off them quickly. Since he is unaccustomed to their hitting in the MICP, the sudden contact during excursion can cause a reflex separation of the teeth.

Check this tooth sensitivity on yourself. Are your anterior teeth out of contact in the MICP? If they are, tap the central incisor sharply with the fingernail of your index finger. Then, with the same force and the same finger, sharply tap a molar that is in MICP contact. You will see immediately that the incisor that is out of MICP contact is much more sensitive to touch than is the molar that is in MICP contact.

It has been shown that a tooth or periodontal ligament loses its sensitivity when it is in trauma. That is why a patient can brux his teeth until he loses them and not be aware of what he is doing. He is so accustomed to the constant tooth contact that he does not know he is bruxing, and he does not know that his teeth have become mobile.

However, forces or impulses less common are easily noticed. Have you ever unexpectedly bitten on a cherry pit? What happened? Your jaw flew open reflexly; you did not have to think about it. It was as if you blew a fuse or tripped the circuit breaker, and the reflex action cut off the current and prevented damage.

So it is with all protective reflexes. When an anterior tooth that is not normally in contact is suddenly contacted, as in the beginning of a lateral bruxing jaw movement, it blows a fuse. Once the fuse is blown, the protective reflex immediately jumps into action, and the muscles tend to open the jaws, to pull the teeth apart, back to their status quo. This stops the lateral bruxing movement.

The next consideration is, if the anterior teeth do not touch, will they erupt until they do touch? No. If they are 1/1000 of an inch out of contact in the MICP, normal incising and chewing plus brush contacts in excursive movements will maintain them that distance apart.

Thus, by maintaining the anterior teeth just a hair's breadth out of MICP contact, they can be used for the cold-shower effect that will help to prevent bruxing. Function and feather-light or brush contact during excursive motion will maintain the anterior teeth in a stable position.

WHEN WOULD ANTERIOR TEETH CONTACT IN THE MICP?

Anterior teeth would contact in the MICP if they were to act as posterior teeth. In this case there should be cusp seats or incisor seats created on the lingual surfaces of the upper anterior teeth. Such a situation occurs when there are no posterior teeth or too few posterior teeth or when the posterior teeth have too little periodontal support.

An incisor seat is a ledge placed on the lingual surfaces of the

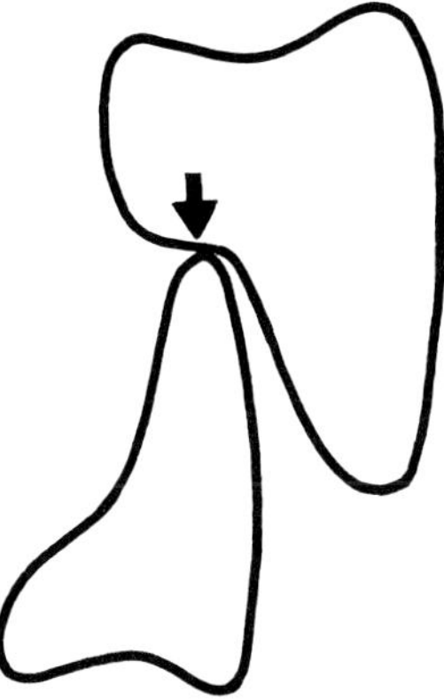

FIG. 67. When an anterior tooth must act as posterior tooth and contact in MICP, an incisor seat (*arrow*) is built. Incisor seat is ledge on lingual surface of upper anterior tooth on which opposing incisal edge rests in MICP. This directs forces as axially as possible.

upper incisors on which the lower incisal edges can contact in the MICP. This better directs the force axially on the incisors (Fig. 67).

Upper cuspids that contact in the MICP should have cusp seats on their lingual surfaces on which the lower cuspids can contact. This better directs the force axially. Treating the lingual surfaces of the upper anterior teeth in this fashion very often requires pin onlays or crowns.

What about the extreme overbite situation, in which the lower anterior teeth occlude with the anterior portion of the palate and the anterior teeth are deprived of their usual function? To treat this condition without orthodontics, simply shorten the lower anterior teeth by grinding their incisal edges. To prevent the lower anterior teeth from erupting, a bite guard must be worn by the patient for a few hours a day, usually during sleep.

SELF-EVALUATION

1. How should the anterior teeth contact in the MICP?

2. What is the cold-shower effect?

3. List in sequence the steps for the occlusal adjustment of the anterior teeth.

6

Adjusting to Centric Relation Occlusion by Selective Grinding

Imagine that you have been asked to write a book about how to ride a bicycle. What would you tell the learner? You would probably describe the various parts of the machine and how they work. Next you might discuss the theory of how a cyclist balances as he moves.

Take one of these topics—the balance that a cyclist needs. How would you explain it in writing so that a learner could go out, get on his bike, and pedal away? The more you would elaborate on this neuromuscular topic, the more complex it would seem and the more discouraged the pupil would become. Yet everyone who cycles knows that the basic skills of cycling are easy to learn.

Occlusal adjustment is not as easy to learn as riding a bike is, but with practice and experience you will learn it. Our problem is to keep our explanations simple and encouraging, without omitting any important information. Your job is to start practicing and gaining experience.

We adjust an occlusion when there is evidence of occlusal restraint that could, in our judgment, result in the loss of teeth. Naturally, if the patient is 80 or 90 years old and has good periodontal support around his teeth, we would not adjust his occlusion unless he was uncomfortable.

The signs that would move us to do occlusal adjustments are fremitus, mobility, and facets. Generally, we would adjust the teeth of most people with these signs. Very often occlusal adjustment by selective grinding is reserved for older people with periodontal breakdown. However, we would prefer to do occlusal adjustments for patients in the late teens and early twenties, as soon as the initial signs become evident.

To do an occlusal adjustment, we have to have a *reproducible reference position* that is physiologically acceptable to the patient and that works clinically. Centric relation is such a position. Therefore, we adjust occlusions to centric relation. This does not mean to imply that centric relation is ideal or normal, but that it is acceptable and it works.

The following is a simple, effective, practical way to do an occlusal adjustment by selective grinding. The adjustment is done to the treatment position of centric relation. The technique is *safe*. We hope that before attempting it you have mastered the techniques of occlusal treatment previously discussed.

WHAT CASES SHOULD YOU SELECT IN THE BEGINNING? Select a patient with a full dentition—24 or more teeth. Select a patient whose slight mobility of the teeth can be demonstrated to him. *Do not* select a patient in pain, with muscle spasm, or with teeth so loose that they are ready to fall out. Select a patient with a centric slip of no more than two millimeters. (Handle the more troublesome situations after you gain experience.)

Dentists continually use some type of articulating paper to adjust their restorations, but they do not as readily attempt an occlusal adjustment by selective grinding. *Jiggling* the patient's jaw to centric relation, *not knowing* exactly where to grind, and *not knowing* exactly what the finished job should look like have caused many dentists to shy away from doing occlusal adjustment by selective grinding.

Furthermore, occlusal adjustment has been discouraged because some patients have developed a "positive occlusal sense." A positive occlusal sense occurs when a patient becomes aware of his teeth and consults the dentist every other day about a different high spot. Sometimes such a patient wanders from dental office to dental office in discomfort, complaining about his bite. He says, "Everything was all right until I had my bite adjusted" or "until I had this bridge made. I've been miserable ever since."

These patients have a legitimate complaint. Centric relation may have been missed, and interferences may have been created by dental treatment. In our experience the most common cause of the difficulty is the loss of holding boundaries in the occlusion. Very often the patients say that it feels as though they have no place to put their jaws. When you hear this complaint, you can be fairly sure that the patient has had his holding boundaries eliminated and has lost his reference. Another way to put it is that the patients do not have a stable MICP, one in which they can repeatedly close the teeth and have them fit.

A positive occlusal sense can also be induced by eliminating lateral restraining contacts on molars and leaving the first millimeter of lateral movement restrained on a bicuspid cuspal incline. This is done by having the occlusal contact one or two millimeters wide buccolingually and having part of this contact on an incline of a cusp. All these problems can be solved or prevented with an understanding of fundamental occlusal principles.

EXAMINATION

Before starting an occlusal adjustment it is important to know the amount and direction of mandibular deflection, that is, the amount and direction of deflection from the position of first tooth contact in centric relation to the maximum intercuspal position.

Why is it important to know this, and how do you find it out? Let us consider first how to discover the mandibular deflection and then why it is important.

The two major obstacles to obtaining centric relation are: (1) the patient's teeth have programmed the neuromuscular system to close to a different position, and (2) it is difficult to get the condyles to their uppermost positions in the glenoid fossae. To overcome these obstacles, the dentist must first eliminate the learned neuromuscular response by getting the patient to relax the mandibular muscles, and after that the dentist (not the patient) raises the condyles to their uppermost position.

Once the condyles are in CR, the dentist closes the mandible to the first light tooth contact. At this first contact, the dentist stops the closure and notes the position. He then asks the patient to squeeze his teeth together. As the patient closes, the teeth slide over one another until they reach the MICP. By watching this slide the dentist can easily detect the extent and the direction in which the teeth deflect the mandible away from CR.

If this deflection is about four millimeters or less, you will be able to do the simplified adjustment described on pages 114–129. But you can do it only if the centric supporting cusps are within a couple of millimeters of their opposing fossae buccolingually when the teeth make initial contact in centric relation. If the centric supporting cusps are far off buccolingually from their opposing fossae, follow the procedure for gross centric adjustment (pp. 111–114): where it is necessary to reshape and move the supporting cusp tips, get the cusp tips as close to opposing fossae as possible, and close the bite back to the original vertical dimension.

Since in most people the MICP is slightly protrusive to CR, the chances are the patient will show a slip from the first CR contact to his MICP. If not, he may be one of those few people whose CR and MICP are the same.

To guide the patient into CR, the dentist first gets the patient to relax his jaw muscles. Tell him, "Let your jaw hang loose. Don't open or close, just hang loose." Once the patient relaxes, the dentist first positions the condyles, and then closes the mandible to the first occlusal contact. To start the manipulation, the patient's teeth should be separated by only a slight distance, a couple of millimeters at most. If the patient opens any wider than that, there is a tendency to tense and resist.

To raise and seat the condyles, the dentist applies an upward and slightly forward pressure at the *angles* of the mandible. At the same time, with his thumb(s), the dentist pulls down the patient's lower lip. By doing this, the dentist allows himself to see the teeth, and also the slight downward pressure on the chin helps rotate the condyles upward and forward. The dentist thus raises the condyles to their uppermost positions and into functional juxtaposition to the articular eminence.

This manipulation can often be done with one hand (Frumker and Arnold), two hands (Mahan and Dawson), or can be achieved by proper jaw jiggling (Ramfjord and Ash).

Learning to guide a patient into centric relation is a necessary skill for you to develop. It is difficult to learn by reading alone. The best way to learn manipulation into centric relation is to befriend a dentist who is expert in this skill and work with him until you also become expert.

For a more complete understanding of centric relation and for a more detailed description of how to manipulate a patient into centric relation, we highly recommend reading Chapter 4 in Dawson's *Evaluation, Diagnosis, and Treatment of Occlusal Problems* and pages 204–211 in Ramfjord and Ash's *Occlusion.* There are also other fine references for techniques for obtaining centric relation (by Guichet, Lucia, Stuart, Long, and so on). We use two or three techniques to double-check ourselves.

Now that you know the how of discovering the amount and direction of the mandibular slide, you need to know the why. If the mandibular teeth retrude in relation to the upper teeth by more than half a cusp or if there is a gross lateral deflection of the mandible (over two millimeters), it may not be possible to adjust the occlusion by selective grinding alone. Orthodontics or rebuilding, or both, may be necessary.

Also, with a large mandibular deflection, if it is possible to adjust the occlusion by selective grinding, you will have to use jaw jiggling in addition to following the simple technique described on pages 114–129.

GROSS CENTRIC ADJUSTMENT

Before you use the method described on pages 114–129, you must reduce a gross discrepancy between centric relation and the MICP to a small one. To determine the discrepancy, you have to guide the patient's mandible into centric relation. When doing so you may find that the lower buccal cusps are lingual to the upper central fossae and the upper lingual cusps are buccal to the lower fossae. In this situation you will also notice that at the initial contact in CR the bite is open a great deal. You must reshape and move the centric supporting cusps so that their tips are as close to their opposing fossae as possible in centric relation. This is where a centric mounting of the study casts comes in handy.

By looking into the mouth and holding the teeth in centric relation contact, you can "eyeball" the grinding of this gross position of the occlusal adjustment. Eyeball grinding means judging the grinding by observation in the mouth and on the models without the aid of articulating paper, ribbon, or wax.

The type of grinding done on supporting cusps is illustrated in Figure 68. It is also possible that, when you place your patient's teeth in centric relation contact, the lower buccal cusps will be buccal to their opposing fossae on one side. Grinding the supporting cusps to eliminate this gross discrepancy is also done by eyeballing.

When you guide the patient into centric relation and have him tap the teeth lightly on the first premature contact, have him point to the tooth that makes the first contact. Then have him squeeze his teeth together and slide from the first contact to his MICP.

If on the side of the first premature contact the mandibular deflection is both protrusive and toward the cheek, the pre-

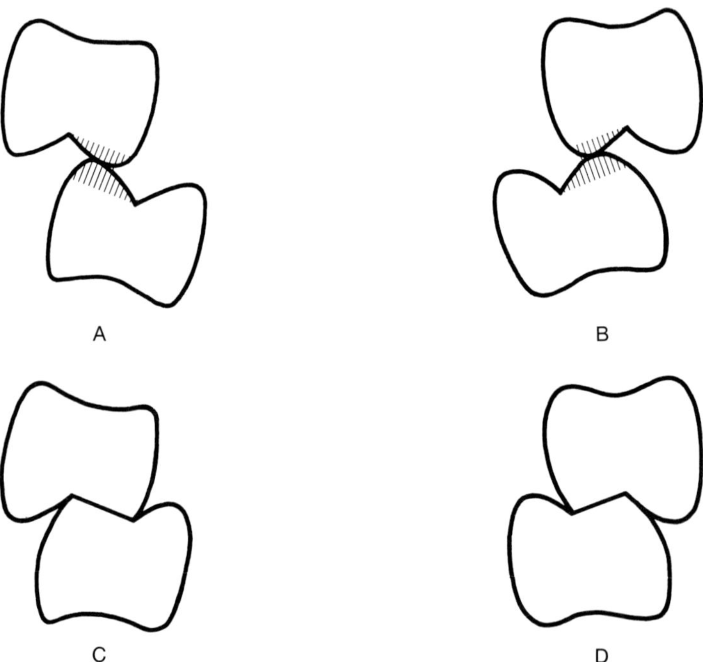

FIG. 68. *A* and *B* represent gross centric premature contacts between centric supporting cusps that hold the bite open in centric relation. In this situation the centric supporting cusps are ground so that their cusp tips are better positioned in line with the center of the opposing teeth and to allow for closing the bite back to the original vertical dimension. The hatched lines show where the grinding is done. *C* and *D* show the result of the grinding.

maturity is on the inner incline of the upper lingual cusp. If the deflection is protrusive and toward the tongue, the prematurity is on the inner incline of the upper buccal cusp of the tooth to which the patient pointed. Once you locate the tooth, mark the first contact with articulating ribbon and do your eyeball grinding.

These gross discrepancies that held the bite so open represent one time that the tips of the supporting cusps are ground and moved. Once the supporting cusps are opposite their opposing fossae (or as close to them as it is possible to reasonably move them) and the bite is still open, you proceed with the dig-in and do no further grinding on the tips of the centric supporting cusps.

Naturally, when the centric supporting cusps begin to get close to their opposing fossae, you should start to use articulating ribbon and stop eyeballing. With these gross centric discrepancies, it is necessary to guide and manipulate the patient's jaw into centric relation contact while articulating ribbon is held between his teeth.

Adjusting the occlusion by jaw jiggling is the same as the method described on pages 117–122 so far as the grinding is concerned. The difference is that you can mark and grind only one or two prematurities at a time when you jiggle the jaw; the method to be described allows you to mark centric prematurities on all the teeth at one time and thus to adjust the occlusion more easily and quickly.

Fortunately, most dentitions show mainly a moderate deflection of the mandible from CR to the MICP, and the vast majority of occlusions requiring adjustment by selective grinding can be adjusted by the simple method described on pages 114–129.

Records are needed before starting the occlusal adjustment. It is important to record tooth mobility. If you do not, you will have no way of proving the merit of your work. Record mobility in millimeters from one to three (Fig. 69). Your recording of mobility may not be exactly like ours, but in time you will become consistent with your own recording, and that is what matters.

Make accurate study casts before the adjustment. You will refer to them numerous times during the grinding of the occlusion. You will also wish to look at them after you have com-

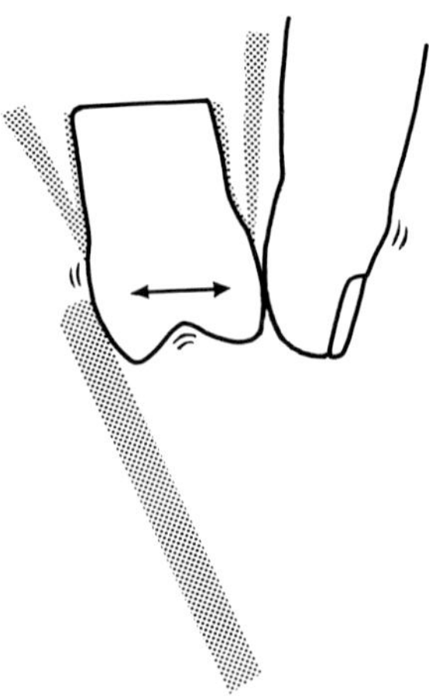

FIG. 69. To test for mobility, hold tooth between instrument and finger as near occlusal surface as possible. Then move tooth buccally and lingually by instrument and finger. Amount of mobility is judged by eye and feel. Most dentists record mobility on a 1-2-3 scale.

pleted the occlusal adjustment in order to compare them to your finished results.

A HINT.   Read the next section on occlusal adjustment until you understand it. Then practice on a cooperative patient who needs an occlusal adjustment. Follow the technique outlined below.

TECHNIQUE

I.   **MARKING THE TEETH.**   On initial examination, salivation characteristics should be noted, whether heavy, normal, or moderate in amount. Or perhaps the mouth is dry.

No premedication to control salivary secretions is necessary for patients with dry mouths. Patients who salivate moderately should take 50 mg. of methantheline bromide (Banthine), a safe drug that is used routinely, one-half to one hour before their appointment. Premedicate heavy salivators with 100 mg. of methantheline bromide. (The drug is contraindicated for patients with glaucoma, pyloric or duodenal obstruction, achalasia, cardiospasm, coronary insufficiency, and cardiac failure.)

You cannot mark wet teeth. Besides premedicating, dry the teeth with cotton rolls or two-inch-square gauze sponges. We use the sponges, others have their patients rub the teeth on cotton rolls. Dry the teeth as best you can.

Next, place heavy blue articulating paper between the teeth and tell the patient to "chop, chop". This command usually keeps the patient from chewing on the paper and makes him smash his teeth together harder. If the patient chops lightly, tell him "harder."

Remove the articulating paper and have the patient hold his mouth open while you get the red articulating ribbon. If he closes and swallows, the teeth will get wet and the markings will be washed away. Remember, you cannot mark wet teeth.

Place the red articulating ribbon between the teeth and again tell the patient to "chop, chop." Place articulating ribbon and paper on both sides of the jaw while the patient chops. If the ribbon or paper is placed on only one side, the patient will have a greater tendency to chew on that side instead of chopping on both sides evenly.

After marking the teeth, have the patient keep his mouth open. If he closes or swallows, you must start all over again since some of the occlusal markings will almost certainly be lost.

Why mark the teeth in this manner? Some dentists use thin blue articulating paper, some use only ribbon, and some use wax. It does not matter to us how you mark the teeth. The end result of the occlusion is what counts. We suggest this system because it works best for us. Wax is also useful, and more will be said about it shortly.

Heavy blue articulating paper is used because it tells where the teeth almost touch. Where the teeth actually do touch, they penetrate the paper and no mark is made. The blue mark is made around the actual contact. Knowing where the teeth almost touch, you can grind the occlusion more rapidly.

Red articulating ribbon is used because it tells where the teeth actually touch. The blue articulating paper and red ribbon used together serve as a verification for a true mark of occlusion between the teeth. With this system the mark of occlusion is a red mark surrounded by a blue mark. When you see this definite mark, you know it is a true record of the occlusion. But the problem with paper and ribbon is that they produce false markings also. False markings are produced because the ribbon and paper is held flat between the teeth. When the patient "chop, chops," the paper and ribbon are dragged across cusps, leaving marks even though there was no contact between the teeth (Fig. 70). When you have used this system for a while, you will easily be able to tell the difference between false and true marks. You can practice by standing in front of the mirror and marking your own teeth. Everything requires practice. When you practice, you will see heavy marks of occlusion on the inner and outer aspects of the supporting cusps. You will also see heavy marks on the inner aspects of the nonsupporting cusps. Next, note the false marks on the tips of the nonsupporting cusps. You cannot help but observe how they differ.

This is the time to practice; there is no sense fumbling in front of a patient. By analyzing the marks on your own

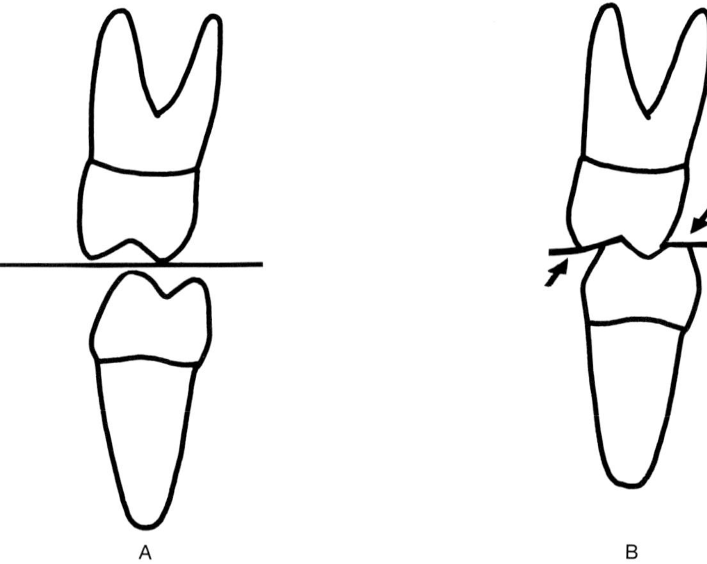

FIG. 70. Articulating ribbon and paper both make false (noncontact) marks on occlusal surfaces. **A,** Ribbon between teeth. **B,** When patient closes, ribbon is smashed between teeth and dragged along tips of nonsupporting cusps (*arrows*). Thus, marks on tips of nonsupporting cusps are false ones. False marks are indefinite, light smudges; true contact marks are definite, heavy, sharp marks. The difference between these marks is discernable.

teeth, you will be able to help patients more quickly. All the marks of occlusion that are described in the following pages can probably be seen in your own or your assistant's mouth. Follow the whole story with your own mouth. Doing so will make occlusal adjustment much more meaningful to you—and more enjoyable too.

A Word About Wax

Wax is the most accurate material for checking occlusal contacts. If you just cannot get the second molars dry and you suspect a contact on the distal marginal ridge, use wax to check yourself. A hole in the wax means occlusal contact, and no hole means no contact. You can be sure with wax, unless a hole was torn in the wax when you pressed it against the teeth while adapting it. No matter what marking system is used, it can be misused. Wax is impractical because it takes too much time, and we rarely use it. (See Figure 71 for hints on using wax.)

II. **GRINDING THE CENTRIC BLOCKING INCLINES.** The mesial inclines of the upper teeth and the distal inclines of the lower teeth that mark are centric blocking inclines. They prevent the mandible from moving distally and reaching centric relation (Figs. 72, 73).

Grind liberally on these marks. Always blend the grinding into the surrounding tooth structure. That means that you will grind a little more than just the mark. *But* do not grind the very tip of a supporting cusp, the very base of a fossa, or the base of a marginal-ridge area that contacts a supporting cusp.

Marginal ridges do have small centric blocking inclines, which will have to be ground if they mark.

A supporting cusp is a cusp that contacts in the MICP so that the mandible is supported by the cusp and the opposing fossa or marginal-ridge area. In most occlusions, the supporting cusps are the lower buccal cusps and the upper lingual cusps. In crossbite occlusions, the supporting cusps are the lower lingual cusps and the upper buccal cusps.

As the first step of the adjustment, simply ask the patient to "chop, chop" on the marking paper and ribbon. Do not try to jiggle the patient's jaw into centric relation and bounce his mandible up and down in centric relation. *We*

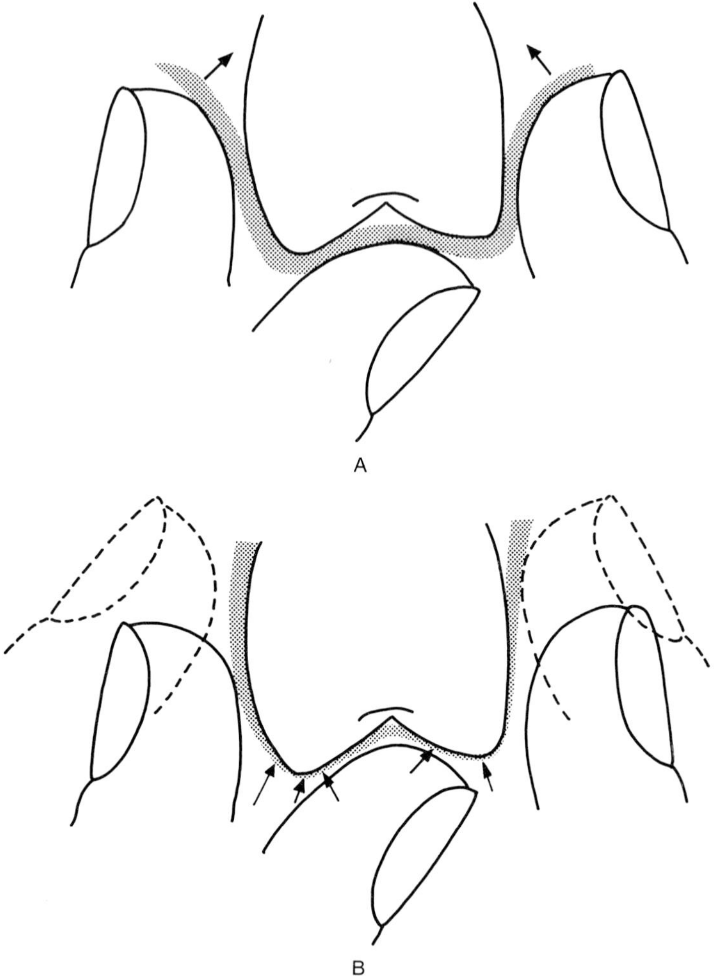

FIG. 71. When adapting wax to teeth, do not stretch or tear it. **A,** Correct adaptation of wax to tooth. Wax is adapted *first* to occlusal surface, then to buccal and lingual surfaces. **B,** Incorrect adaptation of wax to tooth. Wax is adapted first to buccal and lingual surfaces, then to occlusal surface. If handled this way, wax is stretched thin or torn when adapted to occlusal surface. When adapting wax, be careful not to tear it with fingernail.

hope you can visualize any centric blocking incline that marks when the patient closes his teeth in the MICP as a centric interference.

While studying this text, mark your own or your assistant's teeth and pick out the centric blocking inclines. It is a

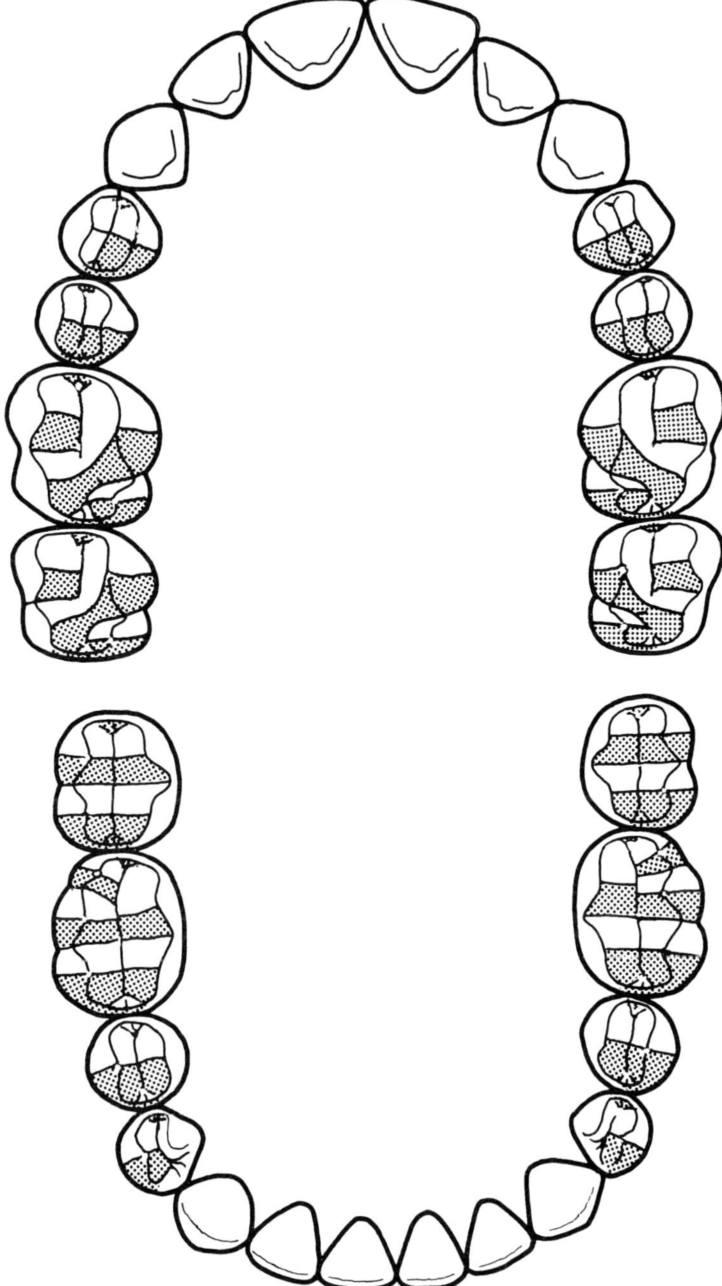

FIG. 72. Holding inclines hold mandible and prevent it from sliding protrusively. They are distal facing inclines of upper teeth and mesial facing inclines of lower teeth (*shaded areas*). Centric blocking inclines block mandible from moving distally. They are mesial inclines of upper teeth and distal inclines of lower teeth (*clear areas*).

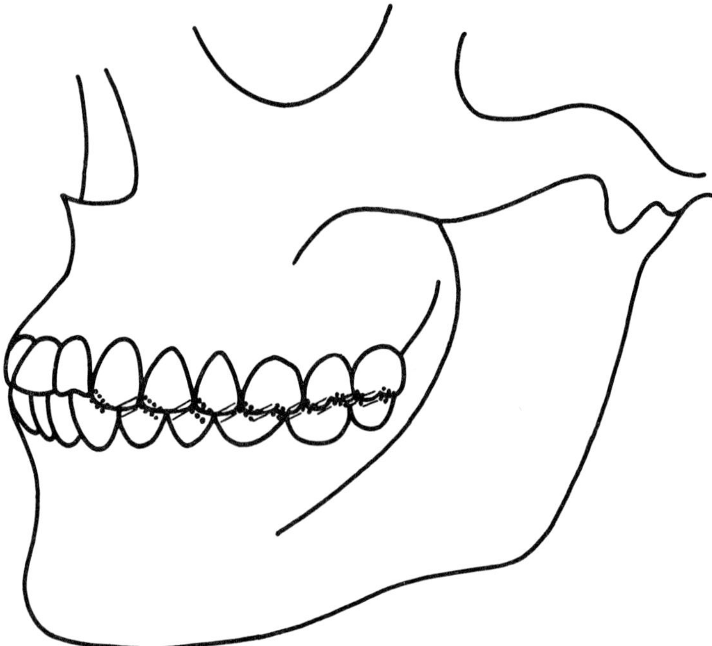

FIG. 73. Sagittal view of centric holding and blocking inclines. Centric holding inclines (*solid lines*) prevent mandible from sliding forward. Centric blocking inclines (*dotted lines*) prevent mandible from moving distally to centric relation. Distal inclines of upper teeth and mesial inclines of lower teeth are centric holding inclines. Mesial inclines of upper teeth and distal inclines of lower teeth are centric blocking inclines.

good idea to study with another dentist who is interested in learning occlusal adjustment. Two heads are usually better than one.

Where to Grind the Centric Blocking Inclines

Grind any centric blocking incline where there is a mark. Grind on the distal inner inclines of the lower lingual cusps and on the mesial inner inclines of the upper buccal cusps. Grind the mesial inner inclines of the upper lingual cusps considerably and the distal inner inclines of the lower buccal cusps to a lesser degree. You will usually grind more on the mesial inner inclines of the upper lingual cusps than you will on the distal inner inclines of the lower buccal cusps.

Grind the mesial outer inclines of the upper lingual

cusps where they mark. Do not grind the distal outer inclines of the lower buccal cusps unless these cusps are severely worn or are buccal to the upper fossae when the teeth are occluded.

Do not grind the tips of the cusps or the bases of fossae or marginal ridges. However, it is important to grind right to the very tips and bases if they mark on their centric blocking inclines. Note that the inner incline of the mesio-lingual cusp of an upper molar, as well as the mesial slope of the oblique ridge, is a centric interference.

When this step is completed, there should be no mark on a mesial incline of an upper tooth or on a distal incline of a lower tooth. *This means that close attention must be paid to the centric blocking inclines associated with fossae and marginal-ridge areas.*

If you leave one millimeter of a centric blocking incline near a fossa in contact, the patient will still have a one-millimeter slip or deflection of the mandible from CR to MICP.

As soon as you have ground all the centric blocking inclines, let the patient rinse his mouth. (Or, since you will be timid and slow at first, perhaps you will have to let the patient rinse before you finish all the centric blocking inclines.) Re-mark and check your grinding until all the marks on the centric blocking inclines have been elim-inated. There should now be no red or blue mark on a centric blocking incline when you mark the teeth.

The elimination of the centric blocking inclines is the hardest part of an occlusal adjustment, but it is not really difficult. Just be sure that you do the job completely.

Let us look at a mistake commonly made during this part of the adjustment, the failure to eliminate the centric blocking incline to its very base (Fig. 74).

More about this part of the adjustment—because the condyles move up and back toward centric relation, the interocclusal space decreases in the molar region and the molars may continue to mark on centric blocking inclines as you grind and re-mark the teeth. You may be surprised to find that the molars are the only teeth that touch after all the centric blocking inclines have been eliminated. Do not be alarmed; it is not unusual to open the bite in the anterior region during this part of the adjustment. The

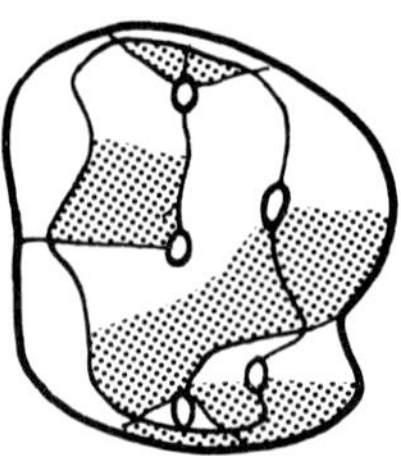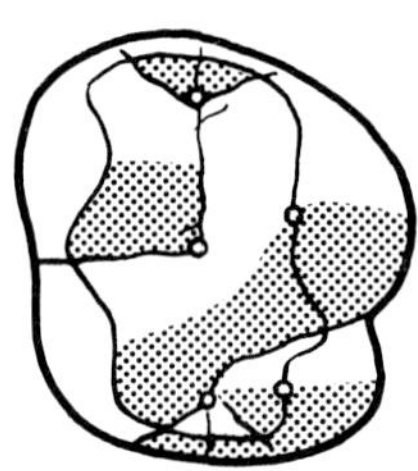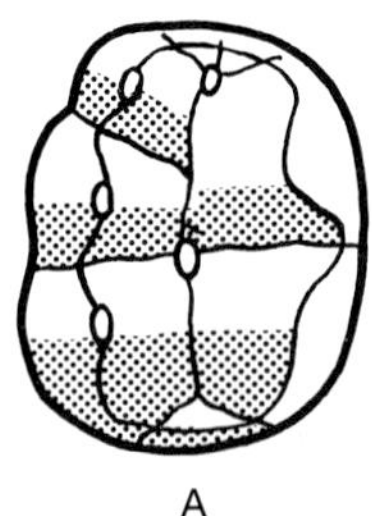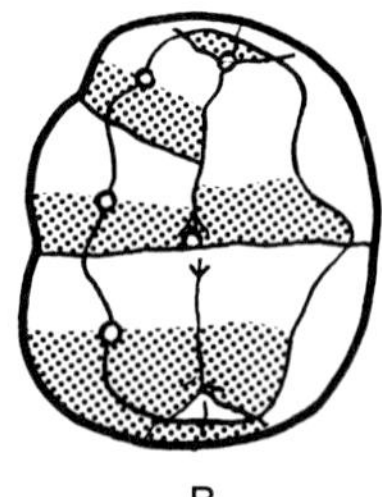

A   B

Fig. 74. **A,** A common mistake. Part of MICP mark is still on centric blocking inclines (mesial incline of upper tooth, distal inclines of lower tooth). Centric blocking inclines must be ground completely out of contact. **B,** Mistake corrected. Centric blocking inclines ground until no marks of contact appear. Marks of contact only in fossae and not extending onto any incline. If centric blocking incline of a marginal ridge is contacted, it must also be ground free of contact.

molars require most of your attention and effort during this initial part of the adjustment.

As the mandible goes distally from a protrusive MICP into centric relation, the condyles follow the articular eminence and move upward and backward. This movement closes the space between the upper and lower ridges in the molar region (Fig. 75). The flatter the plane of occlusion and the larger the move distally, the greater this effect will be. Therefore, as the mandible moves distally toward centric relation, the molars may come into heavy contact and the space between the anterior teeth may open.

III. **GRINDING THE HOLDING INCLINES TO WITHIN ONE MILLI-METER OR LESS OF AN MICP CONTACT.** Grind the holding inclines out of contact except for one millimeter at the base of a fossa or marginal ridge and at the tip of a cusp.

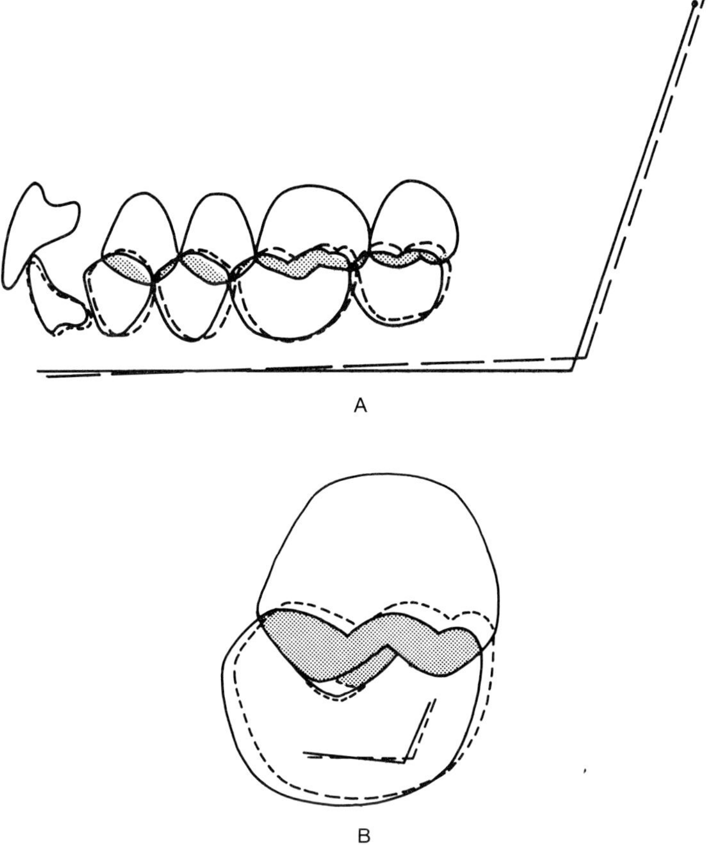

FIG. 75. *A,* Solid line illustrates mandible and teeth in protrusive MICP. Dashed line illustrates mandible and teeth in centric relation (CR). Clear white area inside dashed line of tooth indicates amount of tooth structure that must be removed so that MICP and CR will be the same. Note that as condyle and mandible move up and distally to CR, molars contact first, causing anterior teeth to separate. This is why most grinding will be done on molars and why molars may be the only teeth to touch after centric blocking inclines have been ground free of contact. *B,* Same as *A,* except that *B* focuses on molar teeth.

The holding inclines are not ground liberally. Grind holding inclines very lightly.

To grind the holding inclines, work on the supporting cusps if they are worn and broad. Naturally, do not grind or polish on the tips of these cusps. Grind to within one millimeter of the cusp tip. On an upper supporting cusp, grind the distal slope and on a lower cusp, grind the mesial slope.

If the supporting cusps are not worn, grind on the opposing holding inclines in the fossa or marginal-ridge areas. You may want to split the difference and grind a little off both areas.

The object of this part of the adjustment is to get one millimeter or less of contact between the supporting cusp tips and their opposing fossae, marginal-ridge areas, and (or) holding inclines. This millimeter of contact is in a mesiodistal direction. In a buccolingual direction, the contact should be no greater than a thin pencil line.

The holding inclines must be refined in a buccolingual direction to the width of a thin pencil line. *This is a must to make loose teeth become tight and to prevent tight teeth from becoming loose.* If the final contact is so broad that it has the slightest buccal or lingual slope, it will act as a restraint to the patient and encourage bruxism and tooth mobility.

To insure against restraint, it is imperative that the final mark of occlusion be *no wider than a pencil line* in a buccolingual direction. Keep polishing the buccal and lingual portions of the mark until only the deepest portion remains. When you complete this step you will have a red contact mark up to one millimeter long mesiodistally. Buccolingually, it should be only as wide as a thin pencil line. This mark of occlusion will be between the cusp tip and one of the following: (1) the very deepest part of a fossa, (2) marginal-ridge area, or (3) a holding incline.

It should now be apparent that by eliminating centric blocking inclines to the base of a holding incline, you eliminate deflection of the mandible in a protrusive direction. By refining the contacts in a buccolingual direction to the width of a thin pencil line, you eliminate a deflection of the mandible buccolingually. Dry and mark the teeth again just to make sure you have completed these first two steps of the centric adjustment: (1) elimination of contact between centric blocking inclines and (2) proper grinding and refining of the contacts on holding inclines.

You may want to check the results so far by manipulating the patient's jaw into centric relation. Since you may have missed some centric interferences, this is a good time to place articulating ribbon between the teeth (keep everything dry) to see if any inclines mark. If they do, grind them and recheck your grinding until no centric blocking inclines touch in centric relation.

Do not be surprised if you get contact only between the molar teeth. The next step involves grinding all the teeth back into occlusion. (See page 122 and Figure 75 for the explanation of why the bite is opened during the centric adjustment.)

IV.   **THE DIG-IN.**   If there was much of a centric slip at the start of this adjustment, the bite is now open in the anterior region of the mouth. This is the time for your examination records and models.

If the anterior teeth were touching in the MICP when you began the adjustment, you will want to dig-in the posterior teeth and reduce the vertical dimension until the anterior teeth are again in contact or, at least, within a hair's breadth of contact. If the anterior teeth were not in contact at the start, you will have to refer to the occlusion of the most anterior posterior teeth that were in contact. You must dig-in the posterior teeth until the patient can again contact the same teeth that originally contacted. As you dig-in, you will make centric relation and the MICP one and the same.

The dig-in is similar to the carving of the amalgam restoration that is too high. Remember that on an upper restoration that had not been reduced to proper vertical, you removed the high spot by grinding the mark and distal to it. On a lower restoration, to reduce it to proper vertical dimension, you ground the mark and mesial to it.

As you grind, re-mark the teeth, and check the occlusion, cuspal inclines may come back into contact. If they do, grind them as you did before. Do it along with the dig-in procedure.

Continue the dig-in until the anterior teeth are closed back down to where you originally started the adjustment. Check your examination notes or study models to be sure.

You may ask, "Why are the marks that were so carefully isolated during the initial grinding now being ground during the dig-in?"

The answer is that you cannot do a dig-in until you have isolated the contacts so that only the tips of the supporting cusps contact. Also, it may not be necessary to do a dig-in after the centric slip is eliminated, provided that the bite was not opened in the anterior region.

It is important to dig-in the molars until their contact is slightly lighter than the bicuspids and the bicuspids are hitting slightly harder than the molars. So long as the marks on the molars and bicuspids are even, you cannot be sure that the molars are not hitting harder or prematurely. When the patient marks the teeth for you, they could strike the molars first, spin the mandible around the premature molar contact, and make a mark on the bicuspids. The marks would look as though the contacts on the molars and the bicuspids were even, but actually the marks on the bicuspids would not be true centric contacts and the molars would be hitting prematurely and harder. What happens is that the mandible rotates around the high molar contact, the condyles drop, and, finally, the bicuspids mark just as if they were making true and even centric contacts with the molars (Fig. 76).

Not getting the condyles into their most superior position is also a big problem when manipulating a person's jaw into centric relation. We cannot overemphasize this problem or the need to be sure that the patient hits the bicuspids harder than the molars at the end of the centric

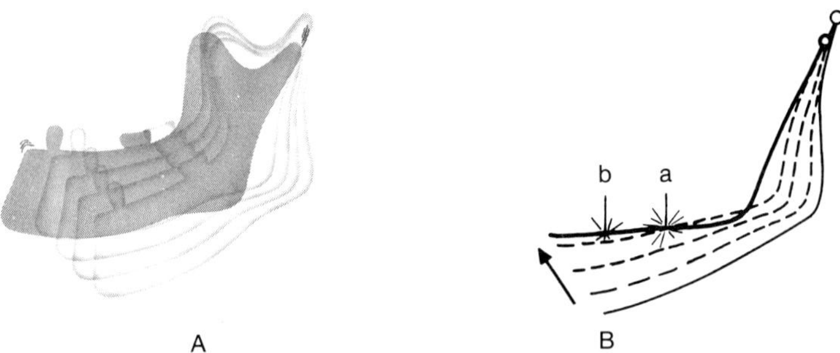

A   B

FIG. 76. ***A,*** Mandible closing in centric relation contacts molar first; condyle drops, and mandible rotates around molar contact and marks bicuspids. Marks look even, but molar is premature. ***B,*** Schematic representation. Asterisk a is premature molar contact. Asterisk b is mark made on bicuspid after mandible rotates around molar. Mark on bicuspid is false since molar is premature and mark on bicuspid is made with condyle pulled down. As long as molar is premature and condyle is pulled down, patient will continue to brux. To avoid this, dig-in molars until mark on molars is lighter than mark on bicuspids. Or simply polish molars out of contact. Molars quickly erupt a hair's breadth back into contact; however, bicuspids left out of occlusion usually do not erupt.

adjustment. We want the patient to feel contact only in the bicuspid region when he chops. At the end of the adjustment, we ask the patient to "chop, chop" and to point to the areas he feels hit hardest. Naturally, we do not want one spot to stand out. If it did, we would adjust it until the patient reports that he feels both sides hitting evenly in the bicuspid area. The molars are a hair's breadth out of contact and they will erupt overnight.

To guard against having the molars hit harder, it is important not to dig-in on the bicuspids until the marks on them are distinctly harder than those on the molars. Caution: A premature contact and a very hard and damaging contact can be much smaller in size than a large smudge. The smudge may be more impressive to the eye, but the small pinpoint mark could be the harder one.

It is not the size of the occlusal mark of contact that determines how heavy or hard the contact is but, rather, the density and appearance of the mark. If you are in doubt, use wax and have the patient "chop, chop."

Now that you have been cautioned about digging-in on the bicuspids, do not forget to eliminate centric blocking inclines any time they mark or reappear on the bicuspids.

Continue the dig-in procedure until the bite is returned either to the vertical dimension that it had when you started or to the vertical you desire.

Remember that during a dig-in procedure you also have the option of shortening the supporting cusp tip. This is often done on upper lingual cusps because they do not wear as much as lower buccal cusps. (The method of doing this is discussed on page 112 and illustrated in Figures 68 and 24.)

If you are digging-in a long upper lingual cusp, it does not make sense to deepen an already deep fossa area. It would be wiser to shorten the upper lingual cusp tip from mesial to distal. Remember that the distal portion of the upper lingual cusp tip is the holding area of the cusp tip; that is why you grind from mesial to distal.

V. **FINAL REFINING.** Polish away any excess contact. Make sure all marks from occlusal contact are as narrow as a thin pencil line buccolingually and no longer than one millimeter mesiodistally. This is the nitty gritty, and it is difficult to do.

Check by jaw manipulation to make sure the patient is in centric relation. If there still is a centric slip, it means that somewhere you may have missed a centric blocking incline. The slip may be slight, but it must be eliminated. Perhaps it is a slight lateral shift that you tried and tried to find but could not. Check the cuspids. Very often it is forgotten that the cuspids can be centric interferences.

If the slip is flat or has no vertical component, there is not a holding boundary coincidental with centric relation. The holding boundary is anterior to centric relation but on the same plane. If this is the case and if the centric slip is slight (one millimeter or less) in a flat, straightforward direction, the result is acceptable so long as the posterior teeth eventually provide the holding boundary at the end of the slide. Having only anterior teeth as a holding boundary for the mandible is not acceptable. The force would be nonaxial and the anterior teeth would be displaced.

Whenever the MICP is anterior to centric relation, be sure to provide freedom for the patient to centric relation. To do this, there cannot be an incline immediately distal to a MICP contact on an upper tooth or mesial to a MICP contact on a lower tooth. This freedom is provided by the cusp seat.

Although we try to make the MICP and centric relation the same, we realize that it is not always feasible when doing an occlusal adjustment by selective grinding alone.

After the centric adjustment is completed, do: (1) the lateral adjustment (Chapter 3), (2) the protrusive adjustment (Chapter 4, posterior teeth; Chapter 5, anterior teeth), and (3) the anterior adjustment (Chapter 5).

After the adjustment is completed, some teeth may not have any satisfactory contacts. Occlusal adjustment by grinding cannot put into the occlusion contacts that were never possible. Occlusal adjustment eliminates deflective or traumatic tooth contacts. It produces the best possible axial loading of the teeth short of restorations.

You must now examine the patient and decide if any restorations are necessary to complete their occlusion. We can assure you that if the patient needs restorations after your adjustment, he needed them before you started. You may get the idea that we think most people need occlusal treatment. We do.

OUTLINE OF THE COMPLETE OCCLUSAL ADJUSTMENT

I. Adjust to centric relation.

1. Mark the teeth.
    Have the patient "chop, chop" into his MICP, first on heavy blue carbon paper, then on red articulating ribbon.

2. Grind centric blocking inclines liberally (the mesial inclines of the upper teeth and the distal inclines of the lower teeth). Grind centric blocking inclines all the way to their bases. Grind holding inclines lightly (the distal inclines of the upper teeth and the mesial inclines of the lower teeth). Grind holding inclines only to within one millimeter of their base. *Do not* grind tips of supporting cusps or bases of fossae and marginal ridges. Centric supporting cusp tips are ground only during the gross centric adjustment, when the centric supporting cusps may be moved bucco-lingually to make them line up with their opposing fossae and marginal ridges.

3. Continue marking and grinding until only the very tips of the cusps and their opposing fossa, marginal-ridge, or central-groove areas contact—and until all contacts are pinpoint in size.

4. If the grinding has resulted in opening the bite anteriorly, do a dig-in until the bicuspids and cuspids are back in contact. The dig-in is accomplished by grinding the contact dot in the cusp seat. Grind dot and distal in upper cusp seats and dot and mesial in lower cusp seats. NOTE: *Only* during a dig-in is the contact dot ground.

5. Once the bicuspids and cuspids are back in contact, continue to dig-in the molars until they contact slightly lighter than the bicuspids.

6. Manipulate the patient into centric relation to make sure there is no longer any centric slip. If because of worn fillings or worn teeth, the patient cannot be ground into a MICP coincidental with centric relation, the slide from centric relation to the holding boundaries should be made short, flat, and straightforward. There should be no incline interfering with centric relation positioning of the occlusion.

7. Have the patient firmly "chop, chop" in centric relation and check all teeth, anterior and posterior, for fremitus. If any is present, grind the tooth until all the fremitus is gone.

II. Adjust lateral jaw movement

1. Eliminate all nonworking-side contact.
Nonworking-side contacts occur between supporting cusps (the lower buccal and upper lingual cusps). CAUTION: In removing nonworking-side contacts, *do not* remove the centric relation contact dot.

2. Select the index tooth.
The cuspid is preferred. If not possible, select the most anterior of the posterior teeth. The index tooth must contact in centric relation (or MICP) and be capable of continuous contact throughout a lateral bruxing jaw movement.

3. Grind the lateral index into the index tooth.
The lateral index is ground smooth. It cannot be bumpy, wavy, or convex. The lateral index must have freedom distally all the way from the patient's protrusive lateral movement to or beyond his border lateral movement. Use the index tooth's marginal ridge as a guide for the correct angle of the lateral index.

4. Create the lateral pathway.
Remove *all* lateral contact from every posterior tooth (assuming that the cuspid is the index tooth) by grinding the inner inclines of the nonsupporting cusps.

During a lateral movement only the index tooth and the incisors can make any contact. CAUTION: In removing lateral contacts, *do not* remove any centric relation contact dots. Once the CR contact dots are established, they are never removed.

5. Check *all* teeth for fremitus during lateral bruxing movement. If any is present, relieve it.

III. Adjust protrusive contacts (assuming that they are on the anterior teeth, as they usually will be. If they are not, follow the instructions on pages 89–92).

1. Adjust the overbite by reducing the incisal edges of the anterior teeth. Follow the smile line in adjusting the incisal edges of the upper anterior teeth.

2. Adjust the CR contacts on the anterior teeth until the contacts are thin lines or small dots.

3. Adjust the incisors in centric and excursive movement to feather-light brush contact by relieving the lingual contacts of the upper anterior teeth. Do not completely relieve the CR contacts yet.

4. Adjust the protrusive contacts until the patient can move his jaw straight forward without any lateral deviation. At this time do all the grinding on the lingual surface of the upper anterior teeth. Do not remove the CR contacts when adjusting protrusive contacts. If the cuspids are the index teeth, try to have their protrusive contacts mark slightly harder than the incisors. If only the incisors contact during the protrusive movement, try to have the marks as even as possible and on as many teeth as possible. Be sure the posterior teeth disclude immediately when a protrusive movement is begun. Adjust the angle of protrusive contact as horizontally as possible while still maintaining posterior immediate disclusion. However, the protrusive angle is not critical as long as the patient has a stable CR.

5. Check all teeth for any fremitus during protrusive jaw movement. If any is present, relieve it.

IV. Remove the CR contacts from all six upper anterior teeth by polishing the centric contact marks on the lingual surfaces of the upper anterior teeth. When you can pull red articulating ribbon between the anterior teeth while the posterior teeth are held firmly together, there will be about 1/1000 of an inch space between the upper and lower anterior teeth.

V. Go back and check:
For fremitus in any position or movement; to make sure all contact dots are pinpoint in size and do not extend buccally or lingually; to make sure all excursive movements are smooth and can easily be done by the patient; to make sure all teeth except the index teeth instantly disclude as soon as any excursive movement is begun.

ADJUSTMENT TO CENTRIC RELATION IN THE YOUNG ADULT

If the dentition is so young that it has not settled in, it should not be adjusted. (However, gross irregularities might be adjusted somewhat.)

If the occlusion requires treatment by altering the occlusal surfaces of the teeth, make sure the problem is not overcarved restorations. If the mouth has restorations with deep anatomy so that occlusal contacts are on inclines, perhaps the overcarved restorations caused or contributed to the occlusal trauma. In this case you will probably have to replace some or all of the restorations after the occlusion is adjusted for freedom.

If the teeth are virgin and supporting cusps are contacting on inclines around fossae, simply adjust the occlusion as suggested. If there is trauma, occlusal treatment is indicated. It is up to you to decide the best way—orthodontics? restorations? grinding? a combination of procedures?

One thing is certain: the last step in *any* occlusal treatment is grinding. You cannot escape it. Either the dentist adjusts the occlusion by grinding or the patient does.

How would one adjust a tipoded or quadrapoded MICP contact to centric relation? First, it must be done carefully.

Grind the centric blocking inclines. If there is a gross protrusive slide of the mandible from the CR to MICP, grind liberally. If there is only a slight slide, grind just a little. Grind, then double-check frequently by having the patient "chop, chop" on the paper and ribbon. Check the mandibular slide from centric relation contact to the MICP. As the slide approaches zero, grind less and less until you have the cusps fitted into the fossae and marginal ridges as well as possible.

Ideally, you finish with tripoded contacts in the fossae. Realistically, you cannot achieve ideal contact. (Nature cannot manage it either.) Practically speaking, though, you will be close enough. Wait a month or two to see if the teeth settle into better contact (Fig. 54). If the contacts cannot be made close, then resort to fillings or orthodontics, or both. Just get the occlusion "fixed up."

The fun of dentistry is the endless opportunity it provides for the dentist to create individual treatment schemes. Happiness is growing toward one's ideals. Not quite reaching them is the fuel that keeps one going and that maintains interest.

A REMINDER: HABITUAL BRUXING IS A DESTRUCTIVE HABIT

If the patient adjusts his own occlusion, he grinds on interfering inclines with opposing supporting cusps. He either destroys the support of his teeth or wears out the teeth.

Why should a patient be allowed to wear out his cusps trying to rid himself of interfering tooth inclines? It is much more reasonable to have a dentist eliminate the interfering inclines with one of his grinding stones. The dentist can selectively grind the interfering areas. The only risk he runs is that of wearing out his grinding stones, and they are easily replaced.

The patient cannot grind his own teeth selectively. He uses his own teeth instead of a grinding stone. He loses two or more times the tooth structure trying to eliminate the trauma. *And,* worst of all, he never does correct the problem; in fact, he aggravates it. The patient wears off the supporting cusps more than he does the interfering inclines. If the dentition can survive, the problem is not eliminated until the teeth are worn in half. But most dentitions do not survive that long; the process usually knocks the teeth out.

SPECIAL CONSIDERATION FOR
MOBILE TEETH

When the occlusal adjustment is completed and all the dots of occlusal contact are as perfect as possible, there is still one small, but critically important, task. Check the mobile teeth to be sure they stand perfectly still when the patient taps his teeth together in centric relation occlusion. Also, make sure the mobile teeth stand perfectly still when the patient moves the mandible from side to side on the index teeth.

Check for fremitus by placing your finger across the buccal surfaces of the upper teeth at the gingival margin while the patient taps and rubs his teeth together. You should not feel any movement of the upper teeth. The way to be sure that the teeth stay perfectly still is to polish the occlusal contacts of the loose teeth slightly out of occlusion. This will give the loose teeth a rest and they will erupt back into occlusion within a week. They will also be tight or, at least, tighter.

Since fremitus on a lower tooth cannot be detected, it is important to polish very loose lower teeth just out of occlusion. If all the teeth are loose, you cannot polish them out of occlusion. Make the occlusal contacts as small as possible and in a week or two lighten the contacts on the teeth that are still very loose. Hopefully, some of them will have tightened.

Secondary occlusal traumatism exists when teeth are loose because they have insufficient periodontal support. The occlusal contacts may be perfect, but there is just not enough bone to hold them. Do not expect teeth with insufficient bone support to become tight. Assuming that the gingivae around these teeth are healthy, the teeth can be splinted so that they are tight. If a tooth is so sick that it adds nothing to the dentition but a liability, extraction is the treatment of choice.

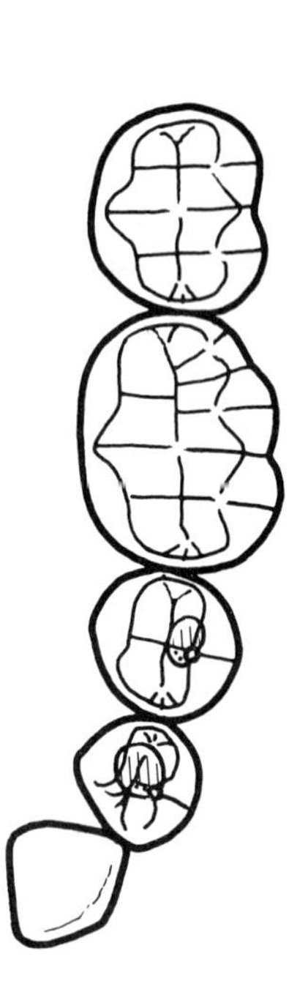

FIG. 77. Centric blocking contacts on bicuspids are represented by vertical lines. Black line around mark indicates area that is ground. A little more than mark is ground so that grinding blends into surrounding tooth structure. Centric blocking marks on bicuspids are mainly on inner inclines of supporting cusps. However, they can and do appear on outer inclines of supporting cusps. In this example, note that mark on upper first bicuspid extends over cusp to mesial outer incline of lingual cusp.

ANOTHER LOOK AT THE GRINDING
OF THE CENTRIC BLOCKING INCLINES

Let us review the grinding to centric relation. While reading the text, look at the marks you made in your own or a friend's mouth.

The initial centric blocking inclines usually seen are the mesial inclines of the upper bicuspid lingual cusps and the distal inner inclines of the lower bicuspid buccal cusps. (In a Class II occlusion, the distal inner inclines of the lower cuspid may hit the upper first bicuspid.) In Figure 77 the initial centric blocking inclines are marked with vertical lines. The circular line shows the area that is ground. More than the centric premature mark is ground so that the grinding blends into the surrounding tooth structure. But note also that the tips of the cusps are not ground, nor are the bases of the fossae.

The next inclines most likely to interfere are the mesial inclines of the oblique ridges of the upper molars. In Figure 78 these inclines are shown as hatched lines. The inclines opposing these are the distal inner and outer inclines of the lower cusps, usually the distobuccal cusps of the lower molars. The circular line indicates the amount of grinding to be done. Note that the distal outer inclines of the lower buccal (supporting) cusps are not ground unless they are worn and flattened or are buccal in relation to their opposing fossae. The opposing upper inclines on nonsupporting cusps are the restraining inclines and so, most of the time, they are ground in preference to the lower outer inclines.

The lower buccal cusps have a greater tendency to strike the inner inclines of the upper buccal cusps during lateral motion. The upper lingual cusps, while they can and do strike the inner inclines of the lower lingual cusps, are less likely to do so because the mandible tips during lateral motion. Naturally, the lower teeth tip also, and so the lower lingual cusps tend to stay

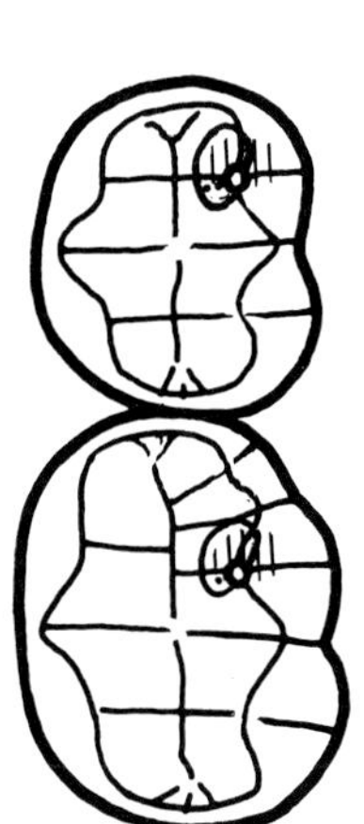

FIG. 78. Centric blocking contacts on oblique ridges of upper molar represented by vertical hatching. Any given patient might make a much smaller or much bigger mark. In worn dentition, mark on oblique ridge might extend from mesiolingual cusp tip all the way to distobuccal cusp tip. If it does, grind everything that marks. Grind centric blocking inclines (mesial inclines of upper teeth and distal inclines of lower teeth) vigorously and completely.

down and away from the upper lingual cusps during lateral motion until the MICP is reached (Fig. 79).

Since the lower buccal cusps have more difficulty escaping and entering the upper arch, more freedom is created by grinding the inner inclines of the upper buccal cusps. Grinding the outer inclines of the lower buccal cusps will not create as much freedom for lateral motion (Fig. 80).

When it is necessary to grind the outer surface of a lower buccal cusp, grind only enough to round off the flat broad outer surface. Do not grind the spot that is directly opposite the fossa or marginal-ridge area that you intend to occlude with the lower buccal cusp.

The next inclines to consider are the inner inclines of the lower lingual cusps (Fig. 81). Grind the distal inner inclines vigorously. Grind the mesial inner inclines (holding inclines) lightly. The circled area shows the typical grinding area.

Now consider the mesial inner inclines of the upper lingual cusps. Grind them as shown by the circled area in Figure 82. The inclines that oppose these are the distal inner inclines of the lower buccal cusps. They, as well as the circled grinding area you must work on to eliminate them, are also shown in Figure 82.

Now the nitty-gritty—the centric blocking inclines of the marginal ridges and fossae. In these areas do not grind the holding inclines, the distal inclines of upper marginal ridges and fossae, and the mesial inclines of the lower marginal ridges and fossae. Do grind the small associated centric blocking inclines, the mesial inclines of the upper marginal ridges and fossae, and the distal inclines of the lower marginal ridges and fossae (Fig. 83).

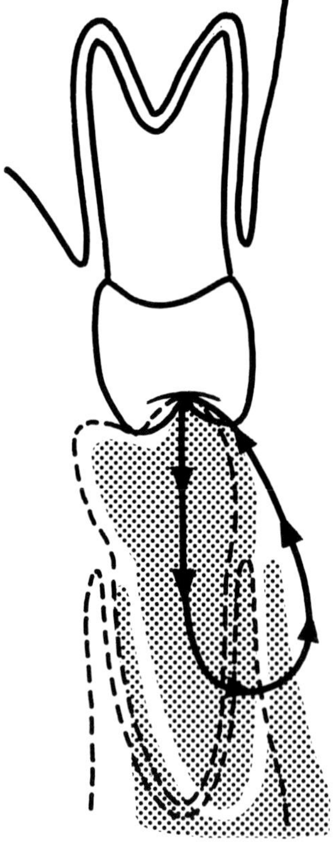

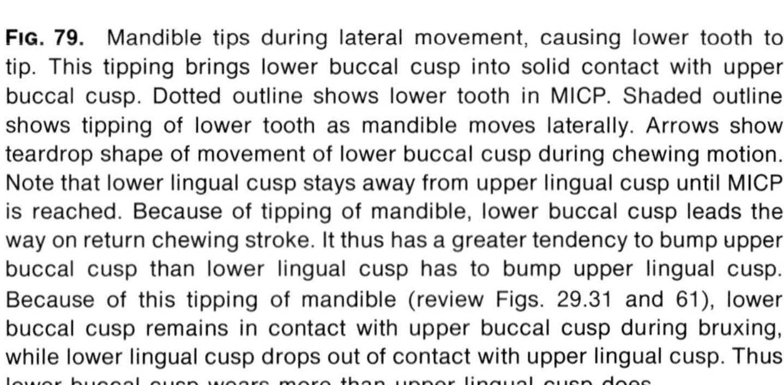

FIG. 79. Mandible tips during lateral movement, causing lower tooth to tip. This tipping brings lower buccal cusp into solid contact with upper buccal cusp. Dotted outline shows lower tooth in MICP. Shaded outline shows tipping of lower tooth as mandible moves laterally. Arrows show teardrop shape of movement of lower buccal cusp during chewing motion. Note that lower lingual cusp stays away from upper lingual cusp until MICP is reached. Because of tipping of mandible, lower buccal cusp leads the way on return chewing stroke. It thus has a greater tendency to bump upper buccal cusp than lower lingual cusp has to bump upper lingual cusp. Because of this tipping of mandible (review Figs. 29.31 and 61), lower buccal cusp remains in contact with upper buccal cusp during bruxing, while lower lingual cusp drops out of contact with upper lingual cusp. Thus lower buccal cusp wears more than upper lingual cusp does.

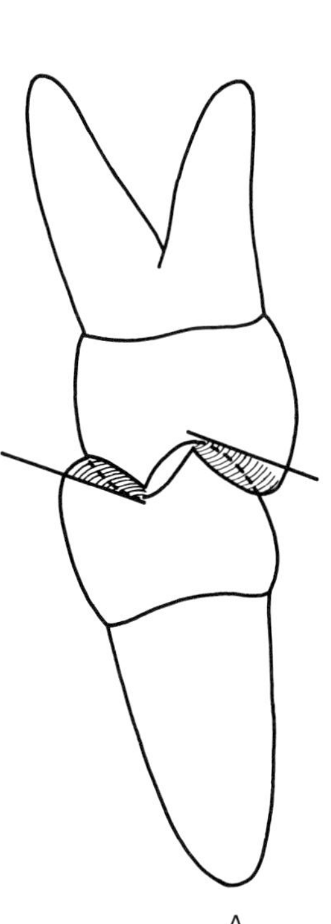
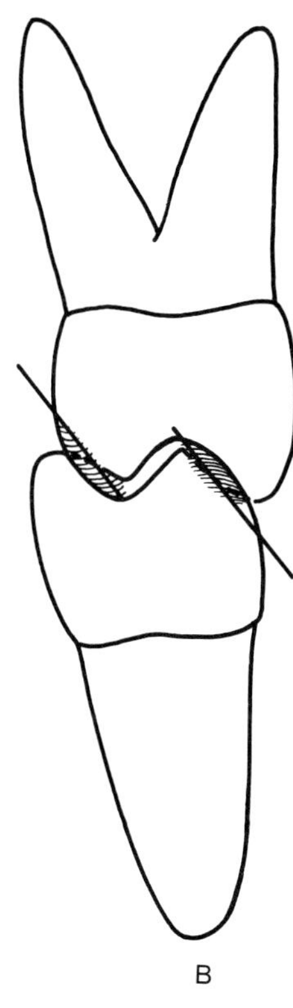

A   B

FIG. 80. *A,* Proper grinding for relief of restraint. Inner inclines of non-supporting cusps have been ground as illustrated by shaded area. Straight lines indicate increased freedom now permitted for supporting cusps. *B,* Improper grinding. Outer inclines of supporting cusps have been ground as illustrated by shaded area. Straight lines indicate lack of freedom permitted for supporting cusps because inner inclines of nonsupporting cusps were not ground.

Key spots that may be missed are the distal inclines of the lower cuspids. In an Angle Class II occlusion, the lower cuspid can occlude with the upper first bicuspid. In this case we usually grind the distal slope of the lower cuspids. You may also grind the mesial inner slope of the lingual cusp of the upper first

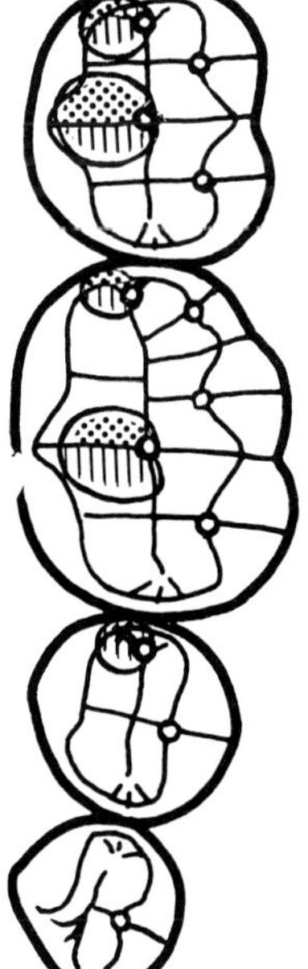

FIG. 81. Typical markings on inner inclines of lower lingual cusps. Part of mark is on centric blocking inclines (*vertical lines*) and part on centric holding inclines (*dotted area*). Grind entire mark except, of course, centric relation contact part of mark. Grind centric blocking inclines more than centric holding inclines. These marks are made by opposing outer inclines of upper lingual cusps. If upper lingual cusp is broad or flattened, grind also outer inclines of upper lingual cusps. When there is a choice between grinding on a nonsupporting cusp or on a supporting cusp, choose the nonsupporting cusp. Why? (Fig. 80.)

bicuspid. In this occlusion, you will notice facets on both of these teeth in the areas mentioned. Get the best relationship you can (Fig. 84).

In Angle Class II occlusion, there is often what is called a *step occlusion*, that is, the occlusal plane of the lower anterior teeth is higher than the occlusal plane of the lower posterior teeth.

Other inclines that must be ground along with the centric blocking inclines are the holding inclines. These inclines are also centric blocking inclines and nonworking-side interferences.

You may ask how these inclines block the mandible from reaching centric relation. The answer is that these inclines on the molars prevent superior positioning of the condyles into centric relation. (Review Figure 75—holding inclines on the molars may also act as centric interferences. To see why they can also act as nonworking-side interferences, review pages 45 and 46.)

Grind all holding inclines to within one millimeter of an MICP contact. Figure 85 illustrates the management of the holding inclines on the molars.

Now that the centric blocking inclines have been ground, wipe all the teeth free of any remaining markings. Dry the teeth and check your work.

It should be obvious that the patient is now better able to close in centric relation. When the teeth are marked again and the patient chops, he will mark centric blocking inclines that were missed during the first grind. Also, he will mark centric blocking inclines where insufficient tooth structure was removed. Check all the marks and adjust as before.

When this step is completed, the only areas that can touch are the tips of the cusps, the bases of fossae, the holding inclines,

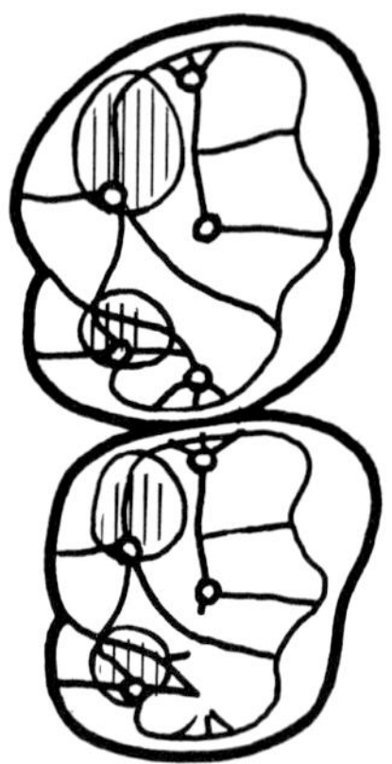

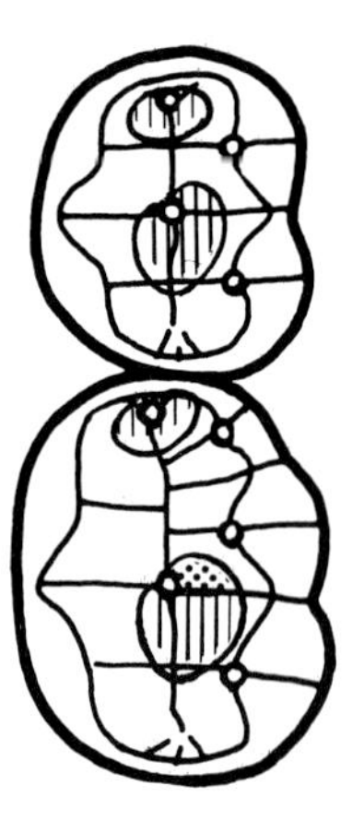

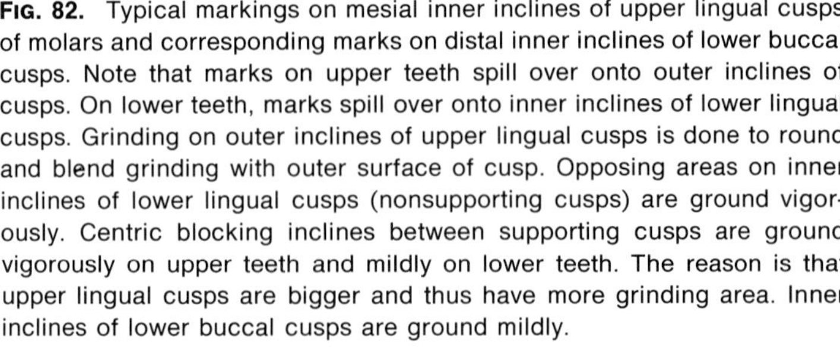

FIG. 82. Typical markings on mesial inner inclines of upper lingual cusps of molars and corresponding marks on distal inner inclines of lower buccal cusps. Note that marks on upper teeth spill over onto outer inclines of cusps. On lower teeth, marks spill over onto inner inclines of lower lingual cusps. Grinding on outer inclines of upper lingual cusps is done to round and blend grinding with outer surface of cusp. Opposing areas on inner inclines of lower lingual cusps (nonsupporting cusps) are ground vigorously. Centric blocking inclines between supporting cusps are ground vigorously on upper teeth and mildly on lower teeth. The reason is that upper lingual cusps are bigger and thus have more grinding area. Inner inclines of lower buccal cusps are ground mildly.

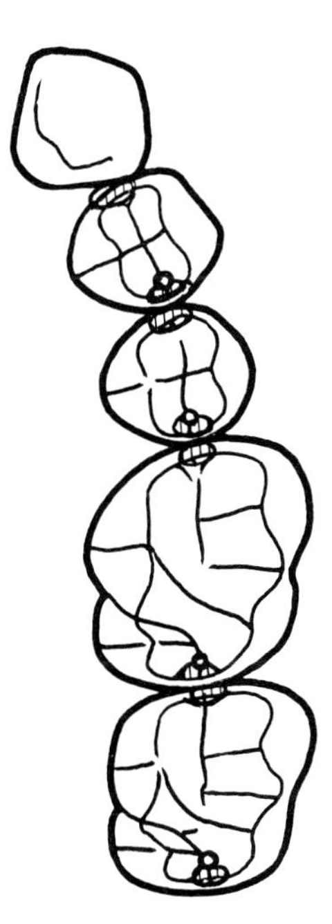

and the holding inclines of marginal ridge areas. All the cuspal inclines are out of contact.

In this discussion of the various areas ground during a centric adjustment, the inclines were isolated and discussed separately. Realize that when you look at a marked tooth in the mouth you see all these inclines marked simultaneously.

Occlusal adjustment is the systematic elimination of contact between inclines of teeth until the mandible is not deflected. You grind the inclines all at once, rather than one at a time, as they were discussed. However, it is important to understand each type of incline contact so that you will know how it deflects the mandible and where and how much to grind.

Proceed with the dig-in and finish the adjustment as previously described (pp. 125–129. Review also Figure 14).

After you finish grinding, check all the teeth for fremitus during occlusion. Place your fingertips over the buccal surfaces of the upper teeth and ask the patient to "chop, chop." There should be no movement of the teeth. Even the loose teeth should stand perfectly still. If they do not, repeat the dig-in until they do not move.

Next, check for fremitus during excursive movement of the mandible. Again, place your fingertips lightly on the buccal surfaces of the upper teeth where they meet the gingiva. Ask the patient to close and rub his teeth lightly in a bruxing movement from side to side and forward. You should not feel any teeth move. If you do, repeat the excursive adjustment on those teeth until they stand still.

The periodontal ligament can heal and the loose teeth can become tight only if the teeth are not subjected to horizontal forces. Recall your patients regularly for occlusal checkups. Touch up the occlusion where necessary.

With a civilized diet tooth wear during mastication does not occur. Consequently, cusps lock and restrain the occlusion (Linghorne 1938, and Murphy 1968). Tooth wear during non-

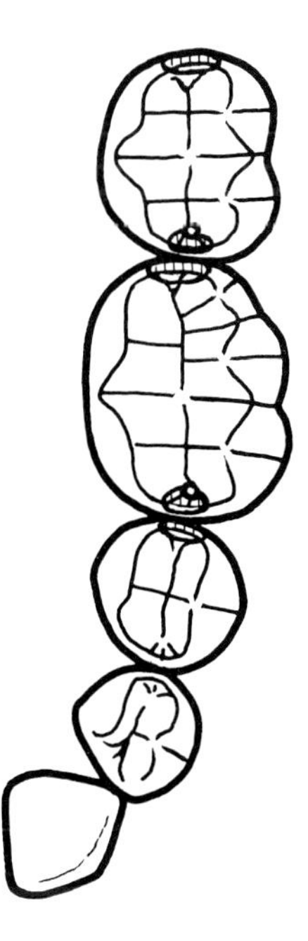

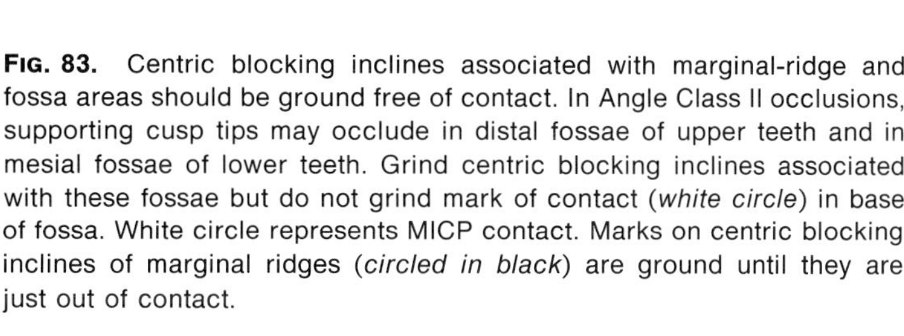

FIG. 83. Centric blocking inclines associated with marginal-ridge and fossa areas should be ground free of contact. In Angle Class II occlusions, supporting cusp tips may occlude in distal fossae of upper teeth and in mesial fossae of lower teeth. Grind centric blocking inclines associated with these fossae but do not grind mark of contact (*white circle*) in base of fossa. White circle represents MICP contact. Marks on centric blocking inclines of marginal ridges (*circled in black*) are ground until they are just out of contact.

functional or bruxing movements does not relieve this locking and restraint, and it is traumatogenic. Thus, most patients show one of the three trouble signs: fremitus, mobility, or wear facets; and early and continuous occlusal treatment is needed. Therefore, preventive occlusal treatment must be included in a preventive approach to dentistry.

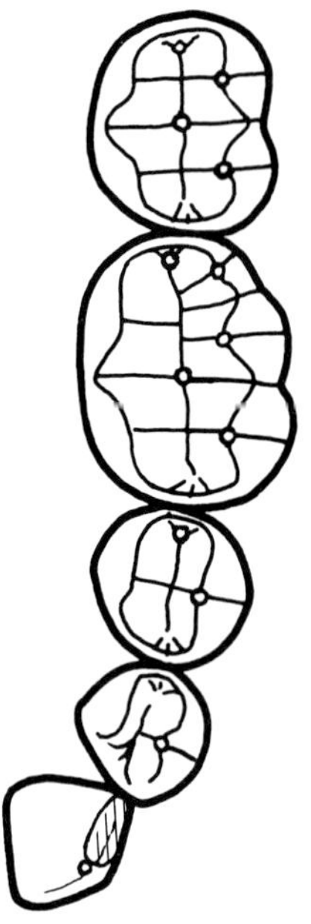

FIG. 84. A common centric interference with Angle Class II occlusal relationship. Distal incline of lower cuspid strikes mesial incline of lingual cusp of upper first bicuspid. Interference is shown in vertical lines, and area to be ground is outlined in black. Note that tip of lower cuspid is not ground. Distal incline of cuspid and mesial incline of lingual cusp of upper first bicuspid are ground. With Class II occlusion, lower cuspid can act as both anterior and posterior tooth. It can occlude with an index tooth and also strike in MICP. Upper first bicuspid or distal of upper cuspid may be used as opposing index tooth, depending on which one contacts better during lateral movement.

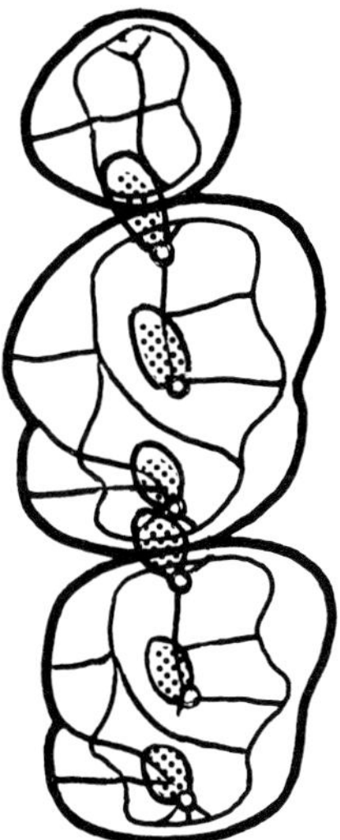

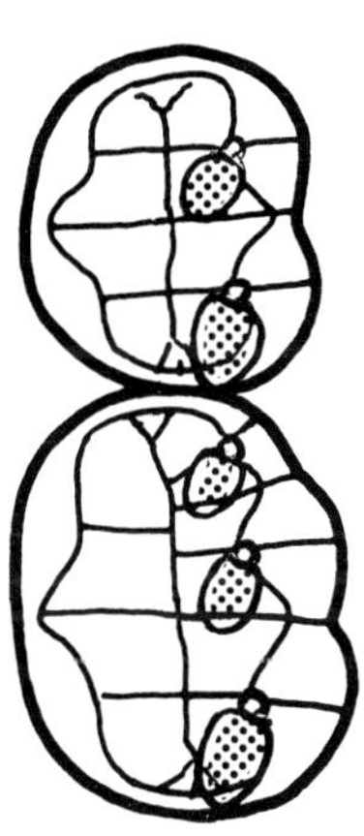

FIG. 85. Holding inclines, especially on molars, may contact when the patient "chop, chops" on red articulating ribbon. Dotted area represents this contact, and area to be ground is outlined in black. Grind holding inclines to within one millimeter of a cusp tip or base of fossa.

Answers to Questions

CHAPTER 2

1. A cusp seat is a therapeutic replacement of a fossa or marginal ridge area.

2. The three parts of a cusp seat are the pinpoint contact, the holding boundary, and the freedom areas.

3. The holding boundary insures that the restoration does not allow the mandible to slip forward.

4. The freedom areas insure that the restoration does not restrain any mandibular movement.

5. The primary contact best axially loads the teeth.

6. In normally related teeth, the primary occlusal contact occurs between the *lower buccal cusp tips* and their opposing fossae or marginal ridges.

7. None. There should be no contact between cuspal inclines. The only occlusal contacts should be the pinpoint primary and stabilizing contacts.

CHAPTER 3

1. In regard to lateral contact, the ideal is no contact. The objective of the lateral pathway is to provide lateral freedom so that the patient will not brux and there will be no lateral contact.

2. Once the MICP contact has been established, a most important rule during the adjustment of lateral interferences is, do not destroy the MICP contacts.

3. On an upper tooth, nonworking-side contacts occur most often on the distal inner inclines of the upper lingual cusps.

4. To relieve nonworking-side contact, most grinding is usually done on an upper tooth.

5. The lateral index is the marginal-ridge area of a normally inclined upper tooth that is contacted by an opposing lower cusp tip during a lateral bruxing jaw movement. If the steeper upper cuspal inclines are contacted instead, as is usual, the lateral index is that part of the upper cuspal incline that is contacted during the lateral movement but that has been so ground that it now forms a plane parallel to the plane of the marginal ridge of the tooth.

6. The index tooth is the upper tooth that has the lateral index on it. It is thus the only upper tooth that can be contacted during a lateral movement.

7. The three criteria for an index tooth are:
   1. It must contact in the MICP.
   2. It should be capable of continuous contact during lateral jaw movements.
   3. It should be firm.

8. A lateral pathway is made by grinding away all the lateral interferences on the remaining teeth so that only the index teeth are capable of contact during lateral movement.

9. The most common error in relieving excursive contacts from the posterior teeth is not grinding all the way to the MICP pinpoint dot, usually leaving .5 to one millimeter of contact buccal or lingual to the MICP dots. The posterior teeth must *immediately* disclude from the MICP dots.

10. Lateral freedom means that there are no interfering inclines that restrain normal and customary lateral movement.

11. Lateral freedom is important because everyone, at one time or another, probably releases muscle tension by bruxing. If

there is lateral freedom, the bruxing will not become a habit and there will be no damage. If there is lateral restraint, the muscles become aware of it, and bruxing becomes a habit and causes occlusal traumatism.

12. The marginal ridges are a landmark that helps determine lateral freedom. The marginal ridges are usually at the proper angles for lateral freedom, assuming a normal axial inclination to the tooth.

13. The three major steps in establishing a lateral pathway are:
    1. Elimination of the nonworking-side contacts
    2. Creation of the lateral index on the index tooth
    3. Elimination of lateral (working-side) interferences

CHAPTER 4

1. Protrusive interferences are cuspal inclines that cause lateral deflection of the mandible during protrusive movement and (or) prevent the most anterior tooth capable of protrusive contact from touching.

2. The cuspal inclines that deflect the mandible laterally during protrusive movement are (1) the mesial inner inclines of the lower lingual cusps and (2) the distal inner inclines of the upper buccal cusps.

3. The best posterior teeth for the protrusive index are the upper bicuspids. Since they are the most anterior of the posterior teeth, the force that can be applied to them is the least.

CHAPTER 5

1. The anterior teeth should not contact in the MICP unless they are worn flat end to end or have an incisor seat on them.

2. When a patient begins a bruxing movement, the anterior teeth that were out of contact in the MICP are contacted

immediately. As a result, there is an abrupt change, like stepping into a cold shower—hence the term *cold-shower effect*. The jaws tend to separate reflexly, and this helps stop the bruxing.

3. The five steps in the adjustment of the anterior teeth are:
   1. Adjustment of the overbite
   2. Adjustment of the MICP contacts to thin lines or dots
   3. Adjustment laterally on the incisors so that there is a brush contact only, making sure there is no fremitus during lateral jaw movement
   4. Adjustment of protrusive movement
   5. Taking the anterior teeth a hair's breadth out of MICP contact by relieving the MICP contact from the lingual surfaces of all six upper anterior teeth.

Glossary

AXIAL FORCE
Force transmitted vertically along the long axis of the root of the tooth.

BENNETT MISS-PATH
Freedom areas of the cusp seats and the lateral index that insure that there will be no occlusal restraint during a Bennett movement.

BENNETT MOVEMENT
Sideward shift of the working condyle during lateral movement of the mandible.

BORDER MOVEMENT
See Posterior border movement.

BORDER POSITION
A most extreme position of the mandible in relation to the maxilla. Centric relation, for example, is a border position because it is the most distal relation of the mandible in relation to the maxilla with the condyles in their uppermost medial position.

BRUXING
Mandibular excursive movement made with the maxillary and mandibular teeth forcibly contacting each other.

BRUXING JAW MOVEMENT
Mandibular excursive movement made with the teeth held firmly together.

CENTRIC BLOCKING INCLINE
Incline that prevents the neuromuscular system from moving the mandible distally into centric relation. The centric blocking inclines are the mesial inclines of the upper teeth and the distal inclines of the lower teeth.

Centric Interference

Tooth-to-tooth contact that prevents a person from positioning his mandible into a centric relation coincidental with the MICP. A tooth-to-tooth contact in the terminal hinge arc of closure that deflects the mandible.

Centric Premature Contact

See Centric interference.

Centric Relation (CR)

Relation of the mandible to the maxilla when the condyles are in their rearmost, uppermost, and midmost position in the glenoid fossa.

Centric Relation Occlusion

Occlusion in which the maximum intercuspal position of the teeth is coincidental with centric relation; that is, occlusion in which the maximum number of holding contacts occur with the mandible in centric relation.

Cusp Seat

Therapeutic replacement of the fossa and marginal-ridge area of a tooth. The cusp seat has three parts:

1. Pinpoint contact
2. Holding boundary, or reference area
3. Freedom areas

Cuspal Incline

Tooth structure radiating apically from the tip of a cusp, between the cusp tip and the base of the cusp.

Dig-In

Reduction of the occlusal contact point on a restoration or tooth that is high, so as to bring the restoration or tooth into equal contact with other teeth, and resulting in the creation of a cusp seat.

Distal Incline

Cuspal incline that faces posteriorly or backward.

Embrasure

A V-shaped space formed by the marginal ridges of two adjoining teeth in contact.

Excursive Movement

Any movement of the mandible to or from its MICP. The movement can be sideward (lateral), forward (protrusive), or both —and also retrusive (backward) if the MICP is protrusive to centric relation.

Facet

Area of tooth surface that is flattened and worn and polished smooth by contact with an opposing tooth; an abraided and polished area on the tooth structure associated with bruxism. The facet can be used as a diagnostic sign of occlusal traumatism.

FREEDOM

Capability of the neuromuscular system to move the mandible to and from occlusal contacts without cuspal inclines interfering with the movement.

FREEDOM AREA

Space around an occlusal contact in which a cusp can move without bumping into a cuspal incline.

FREMITUS

Vibrations in an upper tooth that can be felt by the dentist's fingers when the patient makes a bruxing jaw movement or when he taps his teeth together in the MICP.

HOLDING BOUNDARY

Slight rise in the contour of a cusp seat that holds the mandible in place and prevents it from sliding protrusively. The rise is immediately mesial to and continuous with the contact point of an upper cusp seat and immediately distal to and continuous with the contact point of a lower cusp seat. The holding boundary is also the reference area.

HOLDING INCLINE

Incline that tends to hold the mandible in place and to prevent it from sliding protrusively. The holding inclines are the distal inclines of the upper teeth and the mesial inclines of the lower teeth.

INCISOR SEAT

Ledge on the lingual surface or cingulum of an upper anterior tooth which, when contacted by the incisal edge of an opposing lower anterior tooth, directs the forces as axial as possible.

INCLINE

See Cuspal incline

INDEX TOOTH

See Lateral index tooth and Protrusive index tooth.

INNER INCLINE

Incline of a cusp facing toward the central groove of the tooth. It extends from the cusp tip to the central groove.

INTERFERENCE

See Occlusal interference.

LATERAL BORDER MOVEMENT

See Posterior border movement.

LATERAL CONTACT

Contact between upper and lower teeth during a sideward movement of the mandible.

LATERAL INDEX

Surface or area on an upper tooth that, if contacted by a lower cusp tip during a lateral bruxing jaw movement, will allow the mandible to move laterally without interference. For normally related teeth, this is usually either the marginal ridge of the tooth or a plane (after occlusal adjustment) that is parallel to that of the marginal ridge.

Lateral Index Tooth
Tooth with the lateral index on it.

Lateral Interference
Tooth contacts during a lateral bruxing jaw movement that restrain the mandible from its border path of movement.

Lateral Movement
Movement of the mandible sideward.

Lateral Pathway
Tract of air through which a cusp tip passes during lateral movement. It implies complete freedom of access to the MICP, and from it, during all lateral movements without interference from cuspal inclines.

Mandibular Stability
Occlusal contact position from which the mandible will not slip forward or laterally. The position of mandibular stability should be in harmony with the neuromuscular system.

Maximum Intercuspal Position (MICP)
Relation of opposing occlusal surfaces that provides the maximum intercuspation; Position in which there are the maximum number of occlusal holding contacts; Most stable mandible-to-maxilla intercuspal position.

Mesial Incline
Cuspal incline that faces anteriorly, or forward.

Mobility
Loosening of a tooth associated with alterations of the attachment apparatus.

Nonsupporting Cusp
Cusps that do not contact opposing occlusal surfaces in the MICP. In normally related teeth, the upper buccal cusps and the lower lingual cusps are the nonsupporting ones.

Nonworking Contact
Contact of the cuspal inclines on the nonworking side during a lateral jaw movement. In normally related teeth, nonworking contact will occur between the distal inner incline of an upper lingual cusp and the mesial inner incline of a lower buccal cusp.

Nonworking Side
Side of the dentition where the condyle orbits rather than rotates. It is the side opposite the side that is chewing.

Occlusal Adjustment

Reshaping of the occluding surfaces of teeth to create patterns of tooth form and contact that will be acceptable to the supporting tissues of the teeth and the neuromuscular system.

Occlusal Interference

Tooth contact that deflects the mandible from a normal path of movement or closure.

Occlusal Restraint

Occlusal interference that prevents the mandible from following normal paths of movements or closure. Occlusal restraint causes occlusal traumatism by inducing a bruxing habit in the patient.

Occlusal Traumatism

Force placed on the tooth in excess of that which the supporting structures can withstand. The major cause of occlusal traumatism is the application of horizontally directed forces to a tooth.

Occlusal Treatment

Any alteration in the shape, form, or position of the occlusal surface of a tooth (or teeth) for the purpose of preventing or treating occlusal disease.

Occlusion

Any or all contacts between opposing teeth.

Opposing Tooth

Tooth (or part of a tooth) that is opposite to another tooth or cusp and which will be contacted by that tooth or cusp when the mandible closes and brings the teeth together. An upper tooth that is contacted by a lower tooth when they come together (and vice versa) is the opposing tooth to the other tooth.

Outer Incline

Incline of a cusp facing toward the cheek or tongue. It extends from the cusp tip buccally onto the buccal surface of the tooth or lingually onto the lingual surface of the tooth.

Posterior Border Movement

Lateral mandibular movement that occurs while the mandible is in its most posterior relation to the maxilla. It is the most distal lateral movement the mandible can make in relation to the maxilla.

Premature Contact (Prematurity)

See Centric interference.

Primary Occlusal Contact

The MICP occlusal contact between opposing teeth that best axially loads the teeth. Normally, it is between the lower buccal cusp tip and the upper fossa, marginal ridges, or cusp seat area (see Fig. 5).

PRIMARY OCCLUSAL TRAUMATISM
Condition in which the tooth (or teeth) has sufficient periodontal support to be healthy and firm, but because of occlusal traumatism the attachment apparatus is diseased.

PROTRUSIVE INDEX
Smooth plane on an upper tooth that if contacted by a lower cusp tip or incisal edge during a protrusive jaw movement will be acceptable to the neuromuscular system and will not deflect the mandible laterally.

PROTRUSIVE-INDEX TOOTH
Tooth that has the protrusive index.

PROTRUSIVE INTERFERENCE
Tooth surface that interferes with the forward or return movement of the mandible, thus forcing the mandible to move sideward or to open excessively.

PROTRUSIVE MOVEMENT
Movement of the mandible forward.

PROTRUSIVE PATHWAY
Tract of air through which a cusp tip passes during a forward movement. The term implies freedom of the musculature to move the mandible forward without interfering tooth surfaces' causing a lateral (sideward) deviation or excessive opening of the jaws.

REFERENCE AREA
Slight rise in the contour of a cusp seat that refers and directs the neuromuscular system to the exact place at which the mandible is to be closed and the teeth brought into intercuspation. The neuromuscular system will close the mandible so that the opposing cusp tip contacts the cusp seat at the very base of the reference area. The reference area is also the holding boundary. (See Holding boundary.)

REFINING THE CONTACT DOT
Taking a contact dot that is too large and reducing it to pinpoint size.

RESTRAINT
See Occlusal restraint.

RETRUSIVE FACET
Facet on a centric blocking incline that deflects the teeth from centric relation occlusion. It indicates bruxing between centric relation and the MICP.

SECONDARY OCCLUSAL TRAUMATISM
Condition in which there is insufficient attachment apparatus to hold the teeth firm. Normal occlusal force is therefore traumatic and the tooth cannot become firm without splinting.

Space Maintainer Contact

Non-axial occlusal contact that is assisted by other contacts (proximal contacts) so that the tooth occupies a space and prevents shifting of the rest of the teeth.

Stabilizing Occlusal Contact

MICP contact that assists the primary occlusal contact in preventing tipping of the teeth. It alone does not axially load the teeth as well as the primary contact, but together they stabilize the teeth. Normally, the stabilizing contact is between the upper lingual cusp tip and the opposing fossa, marginal ridges, or cusp seat area (See Fig. 5).

Supporting Cusp

Cusps that contact opposing occlusal surfaces in the MICP. In normally related teeth, the supporting cusps are the lower buccal cusps and the upper lingual cusps. In the normal adult dentition, the supporting cusps contact the fossae and marginal ridges of the opposing teeth.

Working Side

Side, or half, of a dentition toward which the mandible is moved during a lateral jaw movement; the side which, at a given time, is chewing, or the side where the condyle rotates rather than orbits.

Working-Side Contact

Tooth contact on the working side during lateral movement. It occurs between supporting cusps and inner inclines of non-supporting cusps.

Bibliography

Suggested for Further Study

Dawson, P. E.: Evaluation, Diagnosis, and Treatment of Occlusal Problems. St. Louis, Mosby, 1974.
Kraus, B. S., Jordan, R. E., and Abrams, L.: Dental Anatomy and Occlusion. Baltimore, Williams & Wilkins, 1969, pp. 203–269.
Linghorne, W. J.: A new theory of nature's plan for the human dentition. Oral Health 28:525, 1938. *A pioneer work with much food for thought.*
Ramfjord, S. P., and Ash, M. M.: Occlusion, ed. 2. Philadephia, Saunders, 1971.
Reynolds, J. M.: Occlusal wear facets. J. Prosth. Dent. 24:367, 1970.
Stuart, C. E., and Stallard, H.: A Syllabus on Oral Rehabilitation and Occlusion. 2 vols. San Francisco, School of Dentistry, University of California.

Physiology

Butler, J. H., and Stallard, R. E.: Effect of occlusal relationships on neurophysiological pathways. J. Periodont. Res. 4:141, 1969.
Guyton, A. C.: Structure and Function of the Nervous System. Philadelphia, Saunders, 1972. *Read at least Chapters 1, 2, 3, 4, and 14. Then read Chapters 5, 15, and 16—and the remainder according to your interests.*
Jerge, C. R.: The neurologic mechanism underlying cyclic jaw movements. J. Prosth. Dent. 14:667, 1964.
Kawamura, Y.: Neurophysiologic background of occlusion. Periodontics 5:175, 1967.
Kawamura, Y.: Recent advances in the physiology of mastication. In Emmelin, N., and Zotterman, Y.: Oral Physiology. New York, Pergamon, 1972, pp. 163–204.
Mahan, P. E.: Basic mechanisms underlying the diagnosis and treatment of jaw dysfunction. Notes of the annual meeting of the American Institute of Oral Sciences, January 16–19, 1975.

Mahan, P. E.: Clinical application of recent studies of jaw function and innervation. Notes of the annual meeting of the American Institute of Oral Sciences, January 16–19, 1975.

McNamara, J. A., Jr.: The independent function of the two heads of lateral pterygoid muscle. Am. J. Anat. *138*:197, 1973.

Schaerer, P., Stallard, R. E., and Zander, H. A.: Occlusal interferences and mastication: An electromyographic study. J. Prosth. Dent. *17*:438, 1967.

Occlusal Trauma and Its Relation to Periodontal Breakdown and Health

NOTE: We observed many patients in whom the pattern of bone loss must be related to occlusal traumatism in order to be fully explained and understood.

Bassett, C. A. L.: Biologic significance of piezoelectricity. Calcif. Tiss. Res. *1*:252, 1968.

Bassett, C. A. L.: Effect of force on skeletal tissue. *In* Darling, R. E., and Downey, J.: Physical Basis for Rehabilitation. Philadelphia, Saunders, 1971, pp. 283–316.

Becker, R. O.: Stimulation of partial limb regeneration in rats. Nature (London) *235*:109, 1972.

Becker, R. O., and Murray, D. G.: A method for producing cellular dedifferentiation by means of very small electrical currents. Trans. N.Y. Acad. Sci. *29*:606, 1967.

Beerstecher, E., and Bell, R. W.: Some aspects of the biochemical dynamics in the periodontal ligament and alveolar bone resulting from traumatic occlusion. J. Prosth. Dent. *32*:646, 1974.

Chasens, A. I.: The effect of traumatic occlusion on the periodontium and the associated structures, and treatment by selective grinding of the natural dentition. Dent. Clin. North Am. *6*:63, 1962.

Gadd, G. N., and Brown, A. C.: Effect of force on periodontal capillary flow. IADR Abstracts, 596, 1974.

Linghorne, W. J.: Practical occlusion for the general practitioner. J. Canad. Dent. Assoc. *8*:163–165, 1942.

Palcanis, K. G.: Effect of occlusal trauma on interstitial pressure in the periodontal ligament. J. Dent. Res. *52*:903, 1973.

Reider, C. E.: Development of a simplified system for clinical evaluation of occlusal relationships. Part I. Acquisition of information. J. Prosth. Dent. *33*:264, 1975. *This article merits thorough and careful study.*

Reider, C. E.: Occlusal considerations in preventive care. J. Prosth. Dent. *28*:462, 1972.

Shamos, M. H.: The origin of bioelectric effects in mineralized tissues. J. Dent. Res. *44*:1114, 1965.

Simring, M.: Occlusal adjustment—treat or treatment. *In* Ward, H. L., and Gardner, A. F.: A Periodontal Point of View. Springfield, Ill., Thomas, 1973, pp. 68–74.

Stallard, R. E.: Occlusion: a factor in periodontal disease. Int. Dent. J. *18*:121, 1968.

Svenberg, G.: Influence of trauma from occlusion on the periodontium of dogs with normal and inflamed gingivae. Odontol. Revy. *25*:165, 1974. *Although the experiment described (traumatizing the periodontium by wiggling a tooth) is an ingenious one, it has little, if anything, to do with traumatogenic occlusions. There is a need for clinical studies of the relationship between occlusal traumatism and periodontal breakdown.*

Youdelis, R., and Mann, W.: The prevalence and possible role of nonworking contacts in periodontal disease. Periodontics *3*:219, 1965.

How a Tooth Wears because of Function
(AS OPPOSED TO BRUXISM)

Stein, M. R.: The seven ages of a molar. Dent. Survey *14*:1315, 1938.

Tooth Wear

Brodie, A. G.: The three arcs of mandibular movement as they affect the wear of teeth. Angle Ortho. *39*:217, 1969.

Moses, C. H.: Studies of wear, arrangement and occlusion of the dentition of humans and animals and their relationship to orthodontia, periodontia and prosthodontia. Dental Items Interest *68*:953, 1946.

Murphy, T. R.: The relationship between attritional facets and the occlusal plane in aboriginal Australians. Arch. Oral Biol *9*:269, 1964.

Importance of Occlusal Freedom and Prophylactic Occlusal Adjustment

Murphy, T. R.: The progressive reduction of tooth cusps as it occurs in natural attrition, Dental Practitioner *19*:8, 1968.

Restraint, Stress, and Bruxism

Butler, J. H., and Stallard, R. E.: Physiologic stress and tooth contact. J. Periodont. Res. *4*:152, 1969.

Graf, H.: Bruxism. Dent. Clin. North Am. *13*:659, 1969.

Jankelson, B.: Physiology of human dental occlusion. J. Am. Dent. Assoc. *50*:664, 1955.

Lindqvist, B.: Occlusal interferences in children with bruxism. Odontol. Revy. *24*:141, 1973.

Nadler, S. C.: The importance of bruxing. J. Oral Med. *23*:142, 1968.

Powell, R. N.: Tooth contact during sleep: Association with other events. J. Dent. Res. *44:959*, 1965.

Ramfjord, S. P.: Bruxism, a clinical and electromyographic study. J. Am. Dent. Assoc. *62:21*, 1961.

Yemm, R.: A comparison of the electrical activity of masseter and temporal muscles of human subjects during experimental stress. Arch. Oral Biol. *16:269*, 1971.

Bruxing and Tooth Mobility

Hirt, A. A., and Muhlemann, H. R.: Diagnosis of bruxism by means of tooth mobility measurement. Paradontologie *9:47*, 1955.

Muhlemann, H. R.: Ten years of tooth-mobility measurements. J. Periodont. *31:110*, 1960.

Muhlemann, H. R. Savdir, S., and Rateitschak, K. H.: Tooth mobility—its causes and significance. J. Periodont. *36:148*, 1965.

During Certain Functions, the Mandible Moves Distally to Centric Relation

Graf, H., and Zander, H. A.: Tooth contacts in mastication. J. Prosthet. Dent. *13:1055*, 1963.

The Side With the Greatest Lateral Freedom is Preferred for Chewing; a Multidirectional Occlusion is Best

Beyron, H. L.: Occlusal changes in adult dentition. J.A.D.A. *48:674*, 1954.

Mastication Also Requires Lateral Freedom

Adams, S. H., and Zander, H. A.: Functional tooth contacts in lateral and centric occlusion. J.A.D.A. *69:465*, 1964.

Why Use the Cuspid or Most Anterior of the Posterior Teeth as the Index Tooth?

Gosen, A. J.: Mandibular leverage and occlusion, J. Prosth. Dent. *31:369*, 1974.

Force Distribution throughout the Dental Arch

Mansour, R. M., and Reynik, R. J.: In vivo occlusal forces and moments: I. Forces measured in terminal hinge position and associated moments. J. Dent. Res. *54*:114, 1975.

Bennett Movement

Preiskel, H.: Bennett's movement. A study of human lateral mandibular movement. Brit. Dent. J. *129*:372, 1970.
Preiskel, H.: The canine teeth related to Bennett movement. Brit. Dent. J. *131*:312, 1971.

Helping Understand the Cold-Shower Effect

Hannam, A. G., and Matthewes, B.: Reflex jaw opening in response to stimulation of the periodontal mechanoreceptors in the cat. Arch. Oral Biol. *14*:414, 1969.
Sessle, B. J., and Storey, A. T.: Effects of controlled tooth stimulation on jaw muscle activity in man. Arch. Oral Biol. *17*:597, 1972.

Tooth Sensitivity to Load

Crum, R. J., and Loiselle, R. J.: Oral perception and proprioception: a review of the literature and its significance to prosthesis. J. Prosthet. Dent. *28*:215, 1972.

The Smile Line and Phonetics

Guichet, N. F.: The anterior determinants of occlusion. *In* Guichet, N. F.: Principles of Occlusion. Anaheim, Calif., Denar Corporation, 1970, pp. 67–72.
Pound, E.: The mandibular movements of speech and their seven related values. J. Southern Calif. Dent. Assoc. *34*:435, 1966.

Neuromuscular Response to Altered Function

McNamara, J. A., Jr.: Neuromuscular and skeletal adaptations to altered function in the orofacial region. Am. J. Orthod. *64*:578, 1973.

Registering Centric Relation

Long, J. H.: Locating centric relation with a leaf gauge. J. Prosth. Dent. *29*:707, 1973.
Long, J. H.: Occlusal adjustment. J. Prosth. Dent. *30*:706, 1973.

Occlusion and the Temporomandibular Joint

Buhner, W. A.: A headholder for oriented temporomandibular joint radiographs. J. Prosthet. Dent. *29*:113, 1973.
Weinberg, L. A.: Radiographic investigation into temporomandibular joint function, J. Prosthet. Dent. *33*:672, 1975.

The Wide Scope and Importance of Occlusion

Rickets, R. M.: Occlusion—the medium of dentistry. J. Prosth. Dent., *21:39*, 1969. An important article which makes many significant observations.

Sometimes Mandibular Repositioning is Required Before Occlusal Adjustment

Kovaleski, W. C., III, and De Boever, J.: Influence of occlusal splints on jaw position and musculature in patients with temporomandibular joint dysfunction. J. Prosthet. Dent. *33:321*, 1975.
Weinberg, L. A.: Superior condylar displacement: its diagnosis and treatment. J. Prosthet. Dent. *34:59*, 1975.

Centric Relation and Centric Occlusion Do Not Usually Coincide in the Natural Occlusion

Hoffman, P. J., Silverman, S. I., and Garfinkel, L.: Comparison of condylar position in centric relation and in centric occlusion in dentulous subjects. J. Prosthet. Dent. *30:582*, 1973.

The Interplay Between Mandibular Motion, Muscular Activity, and Occlusal Relationships

Krogh-Poulson, W. G., and Olsson, A.: Management of the occlusion of teeth. *In* Schwartz, L., and Chayes, C. M.: Facial Pain and Mandibular Dysfunction. Philadelphia, W. B. Saunders, 1968, pp. 236–249.

Muscle Tension Anywhere Affects the Entire Person

Feldenkrais, M.: Awareness through Movement. New York, Harper & Row, 1972. *Read at least the first 97 pages. Explains the effects of muscle tension and posture on entire body. Is also a superb discussion of the importance of self-education.*
Kraus, H.: Clinical Treatment of Back and Neck Pain. New York, McGraw-Hill, 1970.

Clinical Centric Relation Is Reproducible Regardless of the Patient's Postural Position

Frumker, S. C.: Centric relation and the postural position of the patient. J. Period. *29:*71, 1958.

Occlusal Principles

NOTE: The same principles are applied in different ways by different authors and clinicians. However, with whatever method, when the principles are correctly used, the occlusal treatment succeeds—and that is the basis for the ways we apply occlusal principles.

Abrams, L., and Coslet, J. G.: Occlusal adjustment by selective grinding. *In* Goldman, H. M., and Cohen, D. W.: Periodontal Therapy, ed. 5. St. Louis, Mosby, 1973, pp. 547–598.

Beyron, H.: Occlusal relations and mastication in Australian aborigines. Acta Odontol. Scand. *22:*597, 1964.

Beyron, J.: Optimal occlusion. Dent. Clin. North Am. *13:*537, 1969.

Brown, S. W.: Disharmony between centric relation and centric occlusion as a factor in producing improper tooth wear and trauma. Dent. Digest *52:*434, 1946.

Dawson, P. E.: Temporomandibular joint pain-dysfunction problems can be solved. J. Prosth. Dent. *29:*100, 1973.

DePietro, A. J.: Concepts of occlusion: A system based on rotational centers of the mandible. Dent. Clin. North Am. *7:*607, 1963.

Gibbs, C. H.: Functional Movements of the Mandible. Ph.D. thesis, Case Western Reserve University, Report No. EDC 4-69-24, Medical Engineering Group, 1969.

Guichet, N. F.: Developing Effective Occlusal Treatment Skills. Anaheim, California, 1973.

Guichet, N. F.: Principles of Occlusion. Anaheim, Calif., Denar Corporation, 1970.

Huffman, R. W., and Regenos, J. W.: Principles of Occlusion. London, Ohio, H & R Press, 1969, pp. I-A-1 through I-C-28; 1973, pp. 34–39; 46–58; 387–429.

Ingraham, R.: Occlusion and operative dentistry. Dent. Clin. North Am. *13:*591, 1969.

Kaplan, R. L.: Concepts of occlusion: Gnathology as a basis for a concept of occlusion. Dent. Clin. North Am. *7:*577, 1963.

Kronfeld, M.: Mouth Rehabilitation, St. Louis, Mosby, 1967, pp. 34–39; 46–58; 387–429.

Lucia, V. O.: The gnathological concept of articulation. Dent. Clin. North Am. *6:*183, 1962.

Lucia, V. O.: Modern Gnathological Concepts. St. Louis, Mosby, 1961, pp. 15–50; 110–139; 256–278; 279–313.

Mann, A. W., and Pankey, L. D.: Concepts of occlusion: The P. M. philosophy of occlusal rehabilitation. Dent. Clin. North Am. *7:*621, 1963.

McCollum, B. B., and Stuart, C. E.: A Research Report (Gnathology). South Pasadena, Calif., Scientific Press, 1955.

O'Leary, J. J.: Tooth mobility. Dent. Clin. North Am. *13*:567, 1969.

Posselt, U.: Physiology of Occlusion and Rehabilitation, ed. 2. Oxford, Blackwell, 1968.

Ross, I. F.: Occlusion, a Concept for Clinicians. St. Louis, Mosby, 1970.

Schuyler, C. H.: Freedom in centric. Dent. Clin. North Am. *13*:681, 1969.

Schuyler, C. H.: Fundamental principles in the correction of occlusal disharmony, natural and artificial. J. Am. Dent. Assoc. *22*:1193, 1935.

Schweitzer, J. M.: Concepts of occlusion: A discussion. Dent. Clin. North Am. *7*:649, 1963.

Schweitzer, J. M.: Dental occlusion: A pragmatic approach. Dent. Clin. North Am. *13*:701, 1969.

Stallard, H., and Stuart, C. E.: Concepts of occlusion: What kind of occlusion should recusped teeth be given? Dent. Clin. North Am. *7*:591, 1963.

And, depending on your interests and wishes, you can expand this beginning bibliography a thousandfold.

Postscript

Over the last 12 years or more, we have treated many, many cases of primary occlusal traumatism in which, after occlusal treatment, the teeth have tightened and remained tight and stable for many years.

The signs of bruxing (fremitus, mobility, and facets) disappeared and remained absent. The fact that the loose teeth got firm and remained firm shows that bruxing was no longer habitual. Our students, both dentists and undergraduates in the dental school of the Case Western Reserve University, have had the same experience.

NOTE.   Yours is—and should be—the most important name in your bibliography. Chart carefully patients who have occlusal traumatism (fremitus, mobility, and so on). Take good occlusal records before doing occlusal treatment and again after completing it. Let these records be your own bibliography of your patients' responses to occlusal treatment.

Occlusal Adjustment Supply List

1. Articulating Paper, Blue, Pressure-Controlled (Pulpdent Corporation of America) (Available at local dental supply store)

2. Articulating Paper Plier (Miller-Type) (Union Broach Company) (Available at local dental supply store)

3. Cratex Polishing Wheels

4. 110P and 111P Diamond Wheels. (Available at local dental supply store)

5. Madame Butterfly Silk Dental Tape, Red Record, 40 Inking, 3/4", 10 yds. (ECR Company, Inc., Two Park Avenue, New York, New York 10016)

6. Occlusal Registration Strips (The Artus Corporation, P.O. Box 511, 201 Dean Street, Englewood, New Jersey 07631)